# Childhood Sexuality and AIDS Education

Primary schoolchildren are frequently shielded from education on sexuality and sexually transmitted diseases in an effort to protect their innocence. In countries like South Africa, where AIDS is particularly widespread, it is especially important to address prevention with younger boys and girls as active social agents with the capacity to engage with AIDS as gendered and sexual beings. This volume addresses the question of children's understanding of AIDS, not simply in terms of their dependence but as active participants in the interpretation of their social worlds.

The volume draws on an interview and ethnographic based study of young children in two socially diverse South African primary schools, as well as interviews conducted with teachers and mothers of young children. It shows how adults sustain the production of childhood sexual innocence and the importance of scaling up programs in AIDS intervention, gender and sexuality. It makes significant contributions to the global debate around childhood sexualities, gender and AIDS education.

**Deevia Bhana** is Professor in the School of Education at the University of KwaZulu-Natal, South Africa.

T0347092

# Routledge Critical Studies in Gender and Sexuality in Education

Series Editors Wayne Martino, Emma Renold, Goli Rezai-Rashti, Jessica Ringrose and Nelson Rodriguez

# Childhood Sexuality and AIDS Education
## The Price of Innocence

**Deevia Bhana**

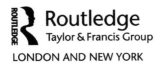

Routledge
Taylor & Francis Group

LONDON AND NEW YORK

First published 2016
by Routledge

2 Park Square, Milton Park, Abingdon, Oxon OX14 4RN
711 Third Avenue, New York, NY 10017, USA

*Routledge is an imprint of the Taylor & Francis Group, an informa business*

First issued in paperback 2017

*Library of Congress Cataloging-in-Publication Data*
Bhana, Deevia.
  Childhood sexuality and AIDS education : the price of innocence / Deevia Bhana. — First Edition.
    pages cm. — (Routledge critical studies in gender and sexuality in education ; 1)
  Includes bibliographical references and index.
  1. Children—Sexual behavior.   2. Sex instruction.   3. Sexually transmitted diseases—Study and teaching.   4. AIDS (Disease)—Prevention.
I. Title.
  HQ784.S45B453 2015
  613.9'51—dc23        2015013566

ISBN: 978-1-138-85300-3 (hbk)
ISBN: 978-1-138-08588-6 (pbk)


Typeset in Sabon
by Apex CoVantage, LLC

**For Adiel and Nikhil**

# Contents

# Acknowledgements

Central to this book are the voices of young children. I owe them so much. This project would not have been possible without the support of the participating schools and their parents and teachers. Over the years I have developed, written and presented ideas of this research, and I would like to thank my colleagues who invited me to present the research and to write with them and who reviewed, listened and sharpened my thinking about childhood sexuality. Special thanks to Bronwynne Anderson, Roger Deacon, Debbie Epstein, Rishi Hansrajh, Vuyo Nkani, Rob Morrell, Lebo Moletsane, Glenda MacNaughton, Claudia Mitchell, Daisy Pillay, Labby Ramrathan and Shakila Singh. I am especially grateful to my friend and colleague Rob Pattman at Stellenbosch University. I was fortunate to have received the Fogarty award in 2007 and 2012, which allowed me to spend part of my sabbatical in the School of Public Health, Columbia University. I am grateful to Quarraisha and Salim Karim of CAPRISA for making this possible. At Columbia I would like to thank Jennifer Hirsch, Carole Vance and John Santelli, as well as Richard Parker and Leslie Roberts.

I was fortunate to present my work at many institutions over the years—Cardiff University; Melbourne University; Teachers College, Columbia University; International Development Studies, Sussex University; New York Law School, Stellenbosch University, North West University—and am grateful for these opportunities. In 2007 I was invited by Carole Vance to present my work in the Programme for the Study of Sexuality, Gender, Health and Human Rights, Columbia University, New York, for which I am very grateful. Between 2008 and 2011, I taught Young Sexualities at Amsterdam University, Summer Sexuality Institute, where this work was presented. To Mike Maxwell, I am so grateful to you. Thank you for bringing this book into shape.

Versions of chapters from this book have been originally published elsewhere. The author and publishers wish to thank the following for permission to reproduce copyright material:

Routledge, Taylor and Francis Group for material from D. Bhana (2007) 'Childhood Sexualities and Rights in HIV Contexts', *Culture, Health and Sexuality,* 9(3): 309–324.

Routledge, Taylor and Francis Group for material from D. Bhana (2008) 'Beyond Stigma? Young Children's Responses to HIV and AIDS', *Culture, Health and Sexuality*, 10(7): 725–738.

Elsevier for material from D. Bhana (2009) ' "AIDS Is Rape" Gender and Sexuality in Children's Responses to HIV/AIDS', *Social Science and Medicine*, 69(4): 596–603.

Routledge, Taylor and Francis Group for material from D. Bhana (2006) 'The (Im)Possibility of Child Sexual Rights in Young South African Children's account of HIV/AIDS", *IDS Bulletin,* 37(4): 64–68.

Routledge, Taylor and Francis Group for material from D. Bhana (2008) 'Sex and the Right to HIV/AIDS Education in Early Childhood', *Journal of Psychology in Africa*, 18(3): 277–282.

Routledge, Taylor and Francis Group for material from D. Bhana (2009) 'How Much Do Young Children Know About HIV and AIDS', *Early Child Development and Care*, 180(8): 1079–1092.

Routledge, Taylor and Francis Group for material from D. Bhana (2007) 'The Price of Innocence: Teachers, Gender, Childhood Sexuality and HIV/AIDS in Early Schooling", *International Journal of Inclusive Education*, 11(4): 431–444.

Routledge, Taylor and Francis Group for material from D. Bhana (2008) 'Discourses of Childhood Innocence in Primary School HIV/AIDS Education in South Africa', *African Journal of AIDS Research*, 7(1): 149–158.

# 1   The Price of Innocence in the Time of AIDS

Johan:[1]  I know how they get AIDS . . . you know like, um (laughter) when you get babies, like you have to like do sort of things . . .

Steven:  Sex stuff . . .

Scelo:  I will only have one girlfriend when I'm older maybe then I would know how to use a condom because now I can't . . .

Vuyo:  If you want to stop AIDS,[2] don't have sex anymore because if you do, you will die early.

In this book I draw attention to the social constructions of gender and sexuality in children's AIDS-related knowledge. I ask, "How do girls and boys, in grade two, aged between seven- and eight-years old, in the South African province of KwaZulu-Natal (the epicentre of the global AIDS pandemic), give meaning to the disease?" "Under what social circumstances are these meanings contested and negotiated?" and "How do adults (teachers and mothers) approach children's AIDS-related knowledge?" To explore these questions in an ethnographic and interview mode, I worked with children in two vastly different race and class settings, one rich and largely white and the other poor and exclusively African.[3] Both contexts are located in the eastern South African seaboard city of Durban, reflecting affluence and adversity, poverty and plenty, and are striking reminders of the effects of history and apartheid. I asked teachers and mothers of children in Grade 2 how they approached children's AIDS-related knowledge. Impelled by AIDS, as the sex-related disease (Weeks 2000), adults told me, "It's difficult for us as Africans to talk about sex to our children," revealing as they did, the paradox of childhood (sexual) innocence and importance of sexuality in AIDS education and prevention (Miedema *et al.* 2015). AIDS not only exposes but also produces the fracture lines of childhood innocence. "Children should not be introduced to this sort of thing at such an early age", adults would tell me—"sex was beyond their age".

To date, few studies place African children, as young as seven and eight, at the centre of investigation, in their own right, for what they can tell us about gender and the constructions of sexuality (Bhana 2007). Nor has there been any attempt to address prevention with younger boys and girls that considers children as active social agents with the capacity to engage with AIDS as gendered and sexual beings (Bhana *et al.* 2006). As Jackson and Scott (2010: 119) note a "childhood free from the shadow of sexuality is thought necessary both to keep children safe and to secure their future sexual health." Children have been short-changed by discourses of childhood innocence. As adults we hide sexuality and silence it (Jackson & Scott 2010). We presume childhood (sexual) innocence, we do not pay much attention to children's pains and pleasures, and we wish childhood sexuality away (Epstein & Johnson 1998). When children express sexuality, we laugh it off as playful, innocent and frivolous (Thorne 1993; MacNaughton 2000; Blaise 2005; Bhana 2013). Childhood innocence is a motif embedded within relations of power and functions as a powerful mechanism of normalization and exclusion producing an exclusive focus on the vulnerable child needing adult protection from sex and sexuality (Kincaid 1998; Egan & Hawkes 2009; Taylor 2010; Clark 2014). In the context of the pressing risk to HIV, we still assume that children are too young to understand sexual knowledge (Silin 1995). Young children remain "too quiet for us to hear, too small for us to see . . . that they fall beneath our threshold of attention" (Tobin 1997: 13). Childhood innocence and the need for child protection justify silence and adult inaction around effective sexuality and AIDS education. The price of innocence, I argue, is the continued inattention and neglect to children's own conceptualisations and experiences of the disease.

By setting in motion the paradox between adult narratives of childhood innocence and children's meanings of AIDS, I aim to oppose everyday common-sense assumptions that question the aptness of putting children and sexuality together (Tobin 1997). Central to my study are seven- and eight-year-old boys and girls, both rich and poor, both black and white, and the complex operation of power. I argue that children interpret, shape and negotiate meanings of the disease as they expand, explore and elaborate on their gendered/(hetero)sexual selves. This process of transgressing, shaping and negotiating the gendered and sexual meanings of the disease is highly complex because boys and girls conceal and reveal sexuality regulating each other as they are regulated by normalised adult versions of childhood innocence. Children do this in ways that express excitement, pleasure and power within a heteronormative context as they defy, negotiate and accommodate dominant ideas of childhood innocence (Renold 2005; Jackson & Scott 2010; Robinson 2013). I emphasise how the epidemic and its sexual route of transmission paradoxically invoke childhood innocence and its instability. At the heart of the paradox, is power. In the chapters that follow and in contrast to adult discourses, I explore girls' and boys' powers, pleasures and anxieties as they uphold/break down childhood innocence, disrupting its hegemony and creating instabilities as they make sense of gender and sexuality in the social construction of AIDS.

In sharpening my analysis, and from the vantage point of poverty and plenty, I focus on the intimate connections between gender, sexuality, race, and class in the social construction of the disease. The selection of two school settings in diverse social contexts in South Africa has been strategic. Children's narratives of AIDS as it relates to the wider social ordering of sexuality, in particular how race, class and gender coalesce around meanings of the disease are key themes in this book. As Farmer (2006: xi) argues, "AIDS is embedded in social and economic structures long in place and that violence, poverty and inequality are the fault lines along which HIV spreads". An understanding of children's AIDS-related sexual knowledge requires a fine-grained analysis of the social, material and discursive forces through which such meanings are made and a critical appreciation of children's agency in promoting and negotiating them. Thus, I pay attention both to the social inequalities through which boys and girls negotiate sexual meanings of the disease and to the active ways in which childhood innocence is promoted and defied. I draw attention to continuities and contrasts among the little social, sexual and cultural worlds of girls and boys and to their pleasures and powers as I show how race, class and gender figure as they shape children's conceptualization of the disease. My hope is that by closely examining what children, in their own right, have to say about the disease, researchers may begin to unravel the knot that has developed in defence of childhood (sexual) innocence and against children's right to sexual knowledge.

In 2003 when I began the qualitative research for this study, approximately 4.2 million people were living with HIV in South Africa. In 2014 the number of people living with HIV has increase to 6.4 million in 2014 with great gender/racial disparities in the rates of infection (Statistics South Africa 2014) and 1.7 million people infected with HIV live in KwaZulu-Natal. In 2014 it was estimated that 15% of Africans are infected compared to 0.3% of whites (Shisana *et al.* 2014). Almost a third of new HIV infections occur amongst young African women between the ages of 15- to 24-year-olds who are more than five to six times more likely to be infected than men of the same age (Karim *et al.* 2014). Much faith has been placed in educational initiatives to provide young people with relevant knowledge and life skills to help them avoid the disease with specific emphasis on gender inequalities and unequal power relation that continue to drive women and girls' disproportionate vulnerability to the disease (Save the Children 2007; UNESCO 2009; Wood & Rolleri 2014; Miedema *et al.* 2015). As Bhana and Singh (2012: 218) argue, "addressing gender inequalities and changing sexual behaviour remain the lynchpin of HIV prevention".

In the world of AIDS, there are increasing efforts to address sexuality in the educational response to the disease:

> Today, in a world with AIDS . . . parents and families play a vital role in shaping the way we understand our sexual and social identities. Parents need to be able to address the physical and behavioural aspects of human sexuality with their children, and children need to be informed and equipped with the knowledge and skills to make

responsible decisions about sexuality, relationships, HIV . . . We have a choice to make: leave children to find their own way through the clouds of partial information, misinformation and outright exploitation that they will find from media, the Internet, peers and the unscrupulous, or instead face up to the challenge of providing clear, well informed, and scientifically-grounded sexuality education based in the universal values of respect and human rights . . . If we are to make an impact on children and young people before they become sexually active, comprehensive sexuality education must become part of the formal school curriculum, delivered by well-trained and supported teachers. Teachers remain trusted sources of knowledge and skills . . . and they are a highly valued resource in the education sector response to AIDS. In the response to AIDS, policy-makers have a special responsibility to lead, to take bold steps and to be prepared to challenge received wisdom when the world throws up new challenges. Nowhere is this more so than in the need to examine our beliefs about sexuality, relationships and what is appropriate to discuss with children and young people in a world affected by AIDS.

(UNESCO 2009: iii)

"We have a choice to make"—leave boys and girls in the early years of life to find their own means and resources to work the puzzle of AIDS/sex/gender/sexuality or "face up to the challenge". By focusing on seven- and eight-year-old children, as they give meaning to AIDS, I take issue with the conceptualization of children as passive and the inattention to gender and childhood sexuality, especially when it concerns children in the early years of life. One of the central aims of this book is to situate sexuality at the centre of how we conceptualise and theorise children's agency in and approach to knowledge of AIDS. By paying attention to children in two socially diverse school settings, I show how race, class, gender and sexuality cut through children's meanings of disease, constricting and setting limits to agency. Through theoretical cross-draughts which brings together different theoretical cross-currents (Therborn 2013), I seek to break from adult scripts of childhood innocence and draw attention to the active ways in which gender and sexuality are produced under striking social conditions of inequalities that cut through children's meanings of AIDS. Overall, a focus on boys, girls and childhood sexuality might contribute to and reconfigure international debates on childhood innocence, agency and AIDS education (Silin 1995; Robinson 2013)—one that conceives of sexuality as central to children's meanings of AIDS but that remains faithful to the effect of material, cultural, symbolic and discursive forces which constrain meaning and agency. In particular, in this book, I summon us as adults to rethink our special responsibility to children in the time of AIDS and to shed our taken-for-granted assumptions about childhood innocence so that we will open our understanding to the creative ways in which children, under strikingly unequal social conditions, work on AIDS, gender, sexuality and relations of power.

In the following section of this chapter, I explore a range of theoretical concepts and perspectives (childhood studies, post-structural feminist theories and theories of structural violence) that collectively contribute to an understanding of children's worlds (as well as the perspectives of adults). Next, I introduce the two sites and focus on researching children, gender and sexuality in the context of AIDS and the implications of conducting research in two vastly different social contexts. Finally, I close with an overview and key summaries of the chapters in this book.

## THEORISING CHILDHOOD SEXUALITY: DISCOURSE, POWER, AGENCY AND VULNERABILITY

> What we see is largely shaped by the frame of the glasses through which we look at the world.
>
> —Therborn (2013: 37)

Childhood is a social category and how adults construct it depends on and is influenced by our frame of glasses (James *et al.* 1998). Instead of seeing childhood as a category of innocence and children as passive and dupes of power, social constructionist perspectives argue that children engage in and work on their everyday circumstances in fluid ways (Kane 2013). Childhood innocence is thus one of many lenses through which we may view children's social worlds. The value of a social constructionist perspective is that it changes the dominating lens from essentialist and biologically determined conceptions of identity to an understanding of children as socially located (Mayall 2002; Blaise 2005; Egan 2013). In developing a theoretical framing for this study I rely on a multidimensional understanding of power. Instead of a fixed meaning of power, power that is fluid and changing allows for variations in making sense of children's complex contextual positioning as gendered and sexual beings. To do this I draw from the sociology of childhood, feminist post-structuralist, queer theorists and structural violence to emphasise gender and sexuality in the construction of agency and the materiality of agency and its social rootedness (Farmer 2004). My attempt at building a "theoretical cross draught" (Therborn 2013) is rooted in and deeply sensitive to, but *not* determined by, the social structures as it permeates gender and sexuality, race, age and class that coalesce in children's articulation of AIDS. The themes of social inequalities and agency pervade this book and are in constant tension with each other.

Throughout this section my aim is not to carve into the already established theoretical literature and debates around childhood, childhood sexuality, agency, and structure because they already exist. The most recent work by Robinson (2013), *Innocence, Knowledge and the Construction of Childhood*, provides comprehensive reviews of theory in relation to childhood innocence, sexuality and agency. There are others, too, including Kane's (2013) *Rethinking Gender and Sexuality in Childhood*, Egan's (2013) *Becoming Sexual: A Critical Appraisal of the Sexualization of Girls*, Parson's (2012) *Growing Up With HIV in Zimbabwe* and Jackson and Scott's (2010)*Theorising Sexuality*, that provide comprehensive reviews of theory. Rather, my intention here is to engage with some of the key theoretical issues and concepts as they have meaning and utility in the operation of power. In the next part of this section, I review some of the main theoretical issues that underlie this study, because they are built up in each of the analysis chapters. The following issues of relevance are discussed here: sexuality and childhood innocence, children as active agents, heterosexuality and the social constitution of sexuality. The section concludes with the tensions between children as gendered and sexual agents and the wider issues of structural violence, which reduce and limit agency.

Sexuality is central to this project and is considered in ways that put post-structuralist feminist theory, queer perspectives and structural violence to work. Sexuality, following Weeks (2000: 163), "pervades the air we breathe". It is fully social and involves sexual desires and practices beyond a simple biological definition of sex (Parker 2009). Sexuality is fluid and contradictory and varies across social contexts. Sexuality is an elastic concept. It stretches through different ideas and feelings. In relation to childhood, instead of plasticity, sexuality is far more rigid. Sexual desires, pleasure and practices are reserved mainly or exclusively for adults, and children are assumed to be uncontaminated by the air we breathe. How do we explain this 'truth' of childhood sexuality? Who can speak the truth about childhood sexuality? Sexuality, as Weeks (2000) suggests, is produced by norms, discourses and regulatory practices and is structured in relations of power. Particularly useful here are the ways in which sexuality functions within a socially organised framework, operating within a regulatory fashion and defining the limits of who can speak the 'truth' about sexuality. A dominant discourse of childhood innocence creates certain 'truths' marked by profound adult–child relations of inequalities and construction of sexuality as inimical to childhood. Once a discourse becomes powerful it is difficult to think and act outside it. Within a particular discourse, only certain things can be said and done. Childhood innocence has become dominant, normalised and the right way of understanding children (Davies 1993). What is right and normal is socially constituted and produced in discourse. Rarely do adults align childhood and sexuality. This is because dominant adult discourses attach power to childhood innocence and at the same time to adults. The norms and practices associated with childhood sexuality include regulation of children's sexual knowledge. The fear that children could lose their innocence if sexuality is raised with them is part of the regulatory discourse and can be seen as a strategic move by adults to limit sexual knowledge. Here sexuality is placed in a binary domain that is dangerous to children and healthy for adults. As Robinson (2013: 8) notes, "childhood innocence is a major force, albeit in the name of protection—in the subjugation of children's lives and functions to maintain relations of power". An abiding concern in this book is the relationship between childhood sexuality and the construction of AIDS as a sex related disease. The discourse of childhood innocence is naturalised, and its harmful effects for others are concealed because of the power that is attached to these meanings. Knowledge about sex and sexuality is restricted by adult discursive constructions and regulations. Children are never outside these discursive environments and relations of power. In appealing to Foucault (1977), knowledge is not neutral but is deeply situated in relations of power and power relations are supported by knowledge (Robinson 2013).

The next important area of value in this book concerns agency and children as active (gendered/sexual) agents. Sexuality, as Weeks (1986) notes, is not given but arises out of struggles, negotiations and agency. Instead of seeing children as sexual dupes, and blanks slates of gender and sexuality, children are agents. As Alanen (1997) notes in understanding the developments in the sociology of childhood:

> Children are treated as speaking, knowing and experiencing subjects, as social actors actively involved in the social worlds they live in, and as interactive agents who engage with people, ideologies and institutions and through this engagement forge a place for themselves in their own social worlds.

As speaking, knowing and experiencing subjects, children are accorded power that is often denied as they are constructed as asexual. In making sense of agency and power I draw from Foucault (1977), who argues that power is not possessed but is something that acts. It is a strategy and involves tactics and where things can be resisted and reversed. Foucault (1980: 98) maintains that power is a locus, "never in anybody's hands, never appropriated". Subjects undergo power as we exercise it:

> When I speak of relations of power, I mean that in human relationships ... power is always present: I mean a relationship in which one person tries to control the conduct of the other ... these power relations are mobile, they can be modified, they are not fixed once and for all ... [they are] thus mobile, reversible, and unstable. It should be noted that power relations are possible only insofar as the subjects are free ... of course, states of domination do indeed exist. In a great many cases, power relations are fixed in such a way that they are perpetually asymmetrical and allow an extremely limited margin of freedom.

Everyone is ensnared by power, but we can modify its grip in specific conditions and as a strategy. The idea that children have power, agency and are active agents is of significance to this book. Adult discourses of childhood innocence appear to be the only way to understand children. In contrast and in line with a post-structural analysis of discourse, power and agency, children are embedded within discursive systems, involving regulation and power where power is not rested on the side of adults only. Children are agents but are also constantly ensnared within power that limits their freedom to express and negotiate sexuality. Of particular concern here are the ways in which boys and girls negotiate power entrenched within 'states of gender and cultural domination'. Feminist post-structuralist thinking allows us to see how particular discourses operate within relations of power that normalise and regulate gender with iniquitous effects. In South Africa there is growing evidence of how schools are places where rigid understandings of masculinity and femininity lead, in some instances, to an "extremely limited margin of freedom", despite variations in masculinity and femininity (Bhana 2008a, 2008b, 2012). Whilst there is recognition of agency, such agency is limited within a discursive environment where the cultural entitlement of male power has diminished opportunities for the expression of girls' agency. I pick this point up again later in the section, but this will be built further in the chapters that follow.

Heterosexuality, as noted by many feminist post-structuralist and queer theorists (Butler 1990), is ordered in unstructured relations of power. Ingraham (1996) for instance defines heterosexuality as an organising principle for gender. The utility of queer theorising is that it questions the sex/gender binary. Butler (1990) uses the term *heterosexual matrix* to explain how heterosexuality is laden with power and taken for granted. Power and privilege occur through a sex/gender binary, where sexual desire is normalised between women and men and other forms of sexuality are repudiated. Of importance is an understanding of queer theory, which recognises and questions the power and privilege associated with heterosexuality because it deepens the understanding of the ways in which gender is constructed. The ways in which boys and girls give meaning to AIDS imbricates with gender and sexuality, where the assumption of sexuality draws from an understanding of desire based on the opposite sex. There is now a growing body of work in childhood studies examining the interaction and the intersection of heterosexuality and gender, particularly by theorists associated with queer theory (Butler 1990; Sedgwick 1990; Thorne 1993; Blaise 2005). In research conducted with young children at school, romantic love, boyfriends and girlfriends, fashion and make-up are now being investigated for their complicity in the heterosexual matrix (see Blaise 2005; Renold 2005). Butler's (1990) work has been pivotal in unhinging the assumed association of sexuality with heteronormativity. The ways in which boys and girls negotiate sexuality are thus highly charged struggles of gendered power as they also give meaning to dominant heterosexuality and enduring forms of gender inequalities that are deeply implicated in the HIV pandemic.

Sexuality attains meaning in social relations requiring attention to context and meanings (Weeks 1986; Jackson & Scott 2010). Sexuality can only be considered in relation to broader social relations through the specific contexts through which sexual practices become meaningful. Corrêa, Petchesky and Parker (2008: 3) add:

> sexuality cannot be understood in isolation from the social, political and economic structures within which is embedded—or without reference to the ideological discourses that give it meaning . . . On the contrary they are shaped by multiple forms of structural violence—social inequalities, poverty and economic exploitation, racism and ethnically based exclusion, gender and sexual oppression, discrimination and stigma, age differentials . . .

There is immense value in understanding sexuality as both negotiated and produced through discursive practices whilst embedded within structural violence—or how power disparities operate. The material conditions set limits to and provide the context of, the everyday world of boys, girls and adults in this study. Materially structured asymmetrical relations of power including race and class divisions do imbricate with and have effects for how sexuality is negotiated and experienced. Of relevance here are the more nuanced ways in which sexuality may be considered. Children are not separate from these relations of power although sexuality and childhood are highly regulated. As Robinson (2013: 13) states,

> Children make choices in their lives but these are always limited by their knowledge and by the specific socio-cultural relations of power that constrain their possibilities, options and agency.

Sexuality is thus conceptualised here in ways that make it possible to understand children as agents with power but in tension with and alongside the social structure. Agency is expressed even in very constrained circumstances. As Jackson and Scott (2010) note, sexuality cannot have any purchase unless it is located within everyday social worlds. Of importance here is how children give meaning to gender and sexuality as they shape and are shaped by the broader social and cultural contexts.

In the final part of this section, I want to augment an understanding of sexuality that takes structure more seriously without abandoning agency, power and active ways in which children are able to express and engage with the social world. I draw from the work of Parker (2001, 2009) and Farmer (2004) to bring together structural violence and agency and to comment further on what this means for an understanding of vulnerability under distressed social conditions. The children (and the adults) in this book occupy different places on the social ladder—with the poor situated in the crucible of poverty and the social inequalities which fuel the spread of HIV. My intention here is to develop an understanding of power and of children's agency that is far more mindful of what it means to navigate conditions of social distress.

Feminist researchers such as Corrêa, Petchesky and Parker (2008) argue for a deeper understanding of structure by drawing from the work of Farmer (2004). Farmer (2004) considers a political-economic analysis of structural factors, which he argues creates vulnerability for the already weakened poor. Farmer argues that gender power inequalities, poverty, economic distress, racism and social marginalisation contribute to oppressive social relations and uses the term *structural violence* to demonstrate this vulnerability. Johan Galtung (1969) coined the term *structural violence* to describe social structures including economic, cultural and political structures that reduce the ability of people to act. Violence, according to Galtung, is not a physical image but is entrenched normalisation and experience of these social structures. The idea of structural violence is linked to oppressive social inequalities. Farmer (2004: 304) posits that

> [s]tructural violence is violence exerted systematically—that is, indirectly—by everyone who belongs to a certain social order . . . In short, the concept of structural violence is intended to inform the study of the social machinery of oppression . . . the impact of extreme poverty and social marginalization is profound in many of the settings . . . In some of these places, there really are social spaces of spirited resistance. Often, however, the impact of such resistance is less than we make it out to be, especially when we contemplate the most desperate struggles and attempt in any serious way to keep a body count. One way of putting it is that the degree to which agency is constrained is correlated inversely, if not always neatly, with the ability to resist marginalization and other forms of oppression . . .

By focusing on HIV and relations of domination, Farmer argues that social structures marked by striking inequalities interacts with unequal relations of power to produce social distress, suffering and illness including HIV. Farmer's analysis grounds material realities and argues that oppression is of political, economic and historical origin. Farmer is sceptical of the ability of people to fight back against what he calls the "infernal machinery" of oppression. Parker argues against Farmer's (2004) mechanistic models of the political economy arguing as feminist post-structuralist theories support a more interactive relationship between structure and agency. Parker (2001, 2009) does, however, recognise the increasing importance of structural violence within conceptualisations of sexuality and argues that inequalities are situated in historical and economical contexts, which shape the possibilities for agency. In other words, sexual cultures can never be understood without gender, race, class and other forms of social inequalities through which sexual relations are organised. In putting structure and agency together Parker notes that the social ordering of relations of sexual contact draws attention to "socially and culturally determined differentials in power" (2009: 260).

Whilst agency and power have been constructed as malleable and plastic, an understanding of children's vulnerability to social conditions, not of their own choosing, remains important. Like structural violence, vulnerability has often been understood as produced by social and economic structures (Kippax *et al.* 2013). The problem with such a conceptualisation of vulnerability is that it assumes that people cannot act until social conditions have been changed which might appear to be an insurmountable task leading to immobilization. Children are, indeed, vulnerable in conditions of ongoing economic misery; however, like structural violence the conceptualisation of vulnerability that excludes the possibility of agency falls short of value in this study. Children are emptied of knowledge, agency and power they may have in conceptualising structural forces as foundational to action. Like Parker (2009), I find that agency and vulnerability are most useful if they are considered together. I pay attention to children, in ways that allow us to suspend an understanding of childhood innocence whilst shedding our assumptions of children as vulnerable victims of social structures demonstrating children as active gendered and sexual beings. I do, however, argue for an understanding of children as both capable of agency and vulnerable in the context of material, symbolic and discursive forces which effectively limit their opportunities and freedoms, diminish agency and call into question the conditions which allow for such inequalities.

## RESEARCHING CHILDHOOD SEXUALITY

The two schools are located in the province of KwaZulu-Natal in the port city of Durban. The province has a complicated history, because of the effects of colonialism and apartheid, and a diverse population. British colonial rule was established in 1843, changing the social and physical landscape of the province. The effects of British colonization are evident in the cultural symbols, the language and with cricket and rugby being dominant sports amongst the white minority in the province. Africans, who make up more than 80% of the population in the province, were historically assigned to work on white farms, and under apartheid black people (including Indian and coloured) more generally were provided with inferior education and unequal resources. The impact of colonization and apartheid has meant fractured and uneven patterns of living and racial/class divisions, which, albeit with change, remain in place. It is part of the pathos of South African history that race and class overlap to the extent that they do, having a negative impact on poor women and children. Today, KwaZulu-Natal has the highest HIV rates in the country, with South Africa regarded as the AIDS capital of the world (Karim *et al.* 2014) and thus locating a study on child-hood sexuality and AIDS education has obvious relevance.

## The Schools: KwaDabeka and Bullwood

The selection of two government schools in varying contexts was not to set one school up against the other but to understand better how meanings of AIDS were socially produced across both the school sites. Purposive sam-pling was used in the selection of schools. This means that the schools were selected based on their typicality and location. KwaDabeka is a quintile 1 school, the designation for the poorest institutions, whilst Bullwood is quintile 5 school, the designation for richer institutions. The quintile system categorises all government schools based on income, unemployment and literacy levels within specific catchment areas of the school (Department of Education 1998, 2006). Children who attend quintile 1 schools are allo-cated a larger subsidy than are children who attend quintile 5. Quintile 5 schools are expected to supplement their state subsidies through the charg-ing of school fees. KwaDabeka is a non-fee-paying school.

The schools are 15-minute drive apart from each other, and despite their proximity they remain vastly unequal in life experiences and resources. The children from KwaDabeka, an African township, are all African and poor. South African townships most vividly illustrate the vast patterns of racial and social inequalities in that they are mainly working class Africans who inhabit what are commonly referred to as one-room *imijondolos* (or 'shacks'), informal settlements combined with newer brick house develop-ments. This population is without income security and has fragile family structures, with reported HIV rates twice as high as those in rural and urban areas (HSRC 2005; Shisana *et al.* 2014). Many children live fragile social contexts with food insecurity and many in single parent (usually female) families. The social context of KwaDabeka bears testimony to the intercon-nected trends of rising unemployment, deepening social inequalities and the increasing scale of gender violence. Underwritten by the legacies of apart-heid and ongoing economic uncertainty, the township location provides contextual specificity in children's account of the sexual and gendered trans-mission of the disease. At KwaDabeka, the total enrolment is 1,181—with approximately 48 to 50 learners in a classroom. The children speak isiZulu as their main language although many understand some English. This is largely because of the proximity of the township to the city of Durban, that many of their parents know and understand English and that English is the main medium of communication from grade 3 to matric in all South African schools.

Bullwood is situated in a wealthy suburban and predominantly white, English-speaking area of Durban. Children come from a context where the HIV statistics indicate that only 0.3% of white South Africans are infected with the disease (Shisana et al. 2014). The school serves about 450 learners, of whom about 25 are African and Indian. The school has approximately 25 children in a classroom. Contemporary South African schooling bears the mark of apartheid, and whilst there have been changes in the racial composition of schools across the country at Bullwood, the changes in racial composition were not as prevalent. The racial mixing in schools is due to a combination of factors, including the financial ability of African families to send their children to former white schools and the availability of public transport to facilitate the movement between rich and poorer areas. Bullwood's particular location, outside of the main public transport lines, made travel to the school difficult for children living in areas outside its residential zone. Bullwood is well-established and affluent, with palatial homes. The school is extremely well resourced and reflective of the context, with much of its money being raised by compulsory fees. Bullwood is an English medium school, and most children have English as their mother tongue, but African children at the school are also very proficient in English.

In total, 174 children composed the study: 64 girls and 55 boys at KwaDabeka and 22 boys and 23 girls at Bullwood. Six of the children at Bullwood were African, and their fees were paid for by a bursary scheme. When I first embarked on this study, the chief focus was children. However, as I worked with children sometimes talking about sexual matters I found them saying, "Please don't tell the teacher." I found myself talking to teachers and asking them questions about what they thought children know and their responses suggested that children were 'not yet ready' for sexual knowledge. As Foucault (1980: 4) writes, if children had no sex, adults (teachers) had "nothing to say about such things, nothing to see, and nothing to know". This also explains the ease with which I received consent by gatekeepers which was in line with this thinking that there was nothing to really know about AIDS from very young children's point of view. While I was beginning to witness the daily transgressions of sexual innocence by young children (through kiss-chase games and everyday conversations about sex) and the hard work they do in negotiating knowing and not knowing sexuality, I began to have discussions with teachers. Five teachers initially were part of the study and I used both group and individual discussions to address the question of children's AIDS-related knowledge. Two more teachers, one from each school, were interviewed later. I draw from these interviews and the conversations I had with teachers in Chapter 6. In other related work I have focused on how teachers taught AIDS (see Morrell *et al.* 2009), but my focus during discussions with teachers was to assess their views about a subject that was controversial and had remained untouched. I also interviewed 21 mothers at both schools during two sets of focus group discussions. At KwaDabeka I interviewed 11 mothers, one group included five mothers and another six. At Bullwood these discussions included five mothers in each discussion; all were white and were by choice stay-at-home mothers. It was not my intention to leave out fathers, but accessing fathers proved to be especially difficult. At KwaDabeka, fathers were either absent or working as migrants outside of the province. At Bullwood, many fathers owned businesses or were in high-profile jobs, making it difficult to ensure a commitment to the interviews.

## Researching From Children's Point of View

The research practices adopted while working with the children in this study were influenced by a deep commitment to putting children first so that they could articulate their views and emotions. I recognised the right of children to set the agenda, introduce and speak authoritatively about issues that they deem to be significant. This kind of work positions itself within a child-centred approach to research, which argues that young children are active agents with the capacity to think, to know and to feel (Frosh *et al.* 2002; Renold 2005). In South Africa, earlier studies have indeed focused attention on children with particular emphasis on teenagers and what it means to grow up in South Africa, especially under adverse conditions but with little or no attention to children as young seven and eight, agency, sexuality and gender, and the methodological implications are limited (Burman & Reynolds 1986; Reynolds 1989; Jones 1993; Barbarin & Richter 2001; Ramphele 2002; Bray *et al.* 2010).

    A close-focus examination of children's meanings was central to this project and in line with feminist post-structural emphasis on power. In order to work closely with children I drew on both ethnographic and interview methods. The fact that children in the two schools have different mother tongues necessitated somewhat different methods of data collection. All interviews with teachers and mothers were conducted in English, but at KwaDabeka I needed the assistance of a translator. My level of proficiency in isiZulu did enable me to break down some of the power relations that shape the research process with children, but I did require assistance with translation. At Bullwood, the conversations were in English. These discussions were conducted in a variety of different settings: out on the grass, in the classroom when teachers gave me permission to work with a group, and during break time. Most children have very few encounters with adults who listen to them in an active and thoughtful way. The research practice in this study was influenced by a deep commitment to the rights of children to articulate their views and emotions and to be considered authorities about issues that they deem significant. I encouraged children to set the agenda. Research drawing from feminist post-structural thinking and the sociology of childhood recognises the right of the child to set the agenda and to determine the way in which the conversations are held, producing evidence of higher competencies in younger children, as Alderson (2007: 2276) notes. Alderson adds that competency is developed through direct social and personal experience and not through age and physical growth. Some of the youngest children can be the most informed and confident about issues that involve them directly within their social contexts. Children in this study felt comfortable to talk about sensitive issues, which they might not have addressed with parents and teachers. This way of working with young children enables freedom of expression and gives them the confidence to ask questions and to refuse to talk and withdraw at their own volition. This research procedure is consistent with the growing tradition of young-person-centred research, which argues that young children are active agents with multiple identities and the capacity to think, to know and to feel (Blaise 2005; Renold 2005; Robinson 2013).

## CONVERSATIONS WITH YOUNG CHILDREN

Like Blaise (2005), Renold (2005) and Thorne (1993) my research put children at the centre of the investigation in ways that maximised their agency. I sat with children at their desks and during break time as they went for sport including swimming lessons. My aim was to hear from children's own account and through their everyday interactions what AIDS might come to mean following unstructured conversational such as in-depth discussions which were organised in varying ways according to the setting or while the teacher had placed children in the class or in lines. At the practical level, classrooms are organised as groups to provide an environment for participation. What this meant for this study is that the groups of children who were seated next to each other (generally between five and six in a group) also made up the groups of children for the research study. At Bullwood desks are arranged in groups of about five or six, and while the teacher has power as an adult (Thorne 1993), the sounds of young children talking, whispering or squealing and their constant movement are a daily feature of the classroom. At Bullwood, before break time, children are allowed to sit outside in groups in the vicinity of their classroom, and it is here that they eat an elaborate lunch that can sometimes consist of sandwiches, juice, snacks, muffins, nuts and raisins while they laugh and chat. I sat with children inside the classroom in their groups as well as outside while they ate snacks. But I also wandered around during the break and talked informally to them. The language of AIDS and sexuality does not sit outside of the everyday social experience. During the course of my conversations with boys a different direction was taken in relation to sport and sporty masculinities. I found this at both schools, and this formed an important area of young masculinities that I have written about elsewhere (Bhana 2008b). At Bullwood, at least once or twice a week, there were cheers in the morning when I arrived, with both boys and girls saying, "Please, please can you sit with us today," or "When are we getting our turn?" Girls in particular would come to me and talk about what they were planning for their birthday parties and whom they would invite. The resource-rich environment meant that children often brought stickers and other toys to school and would conceal them from the teacher and from other peers whom they thought would "tell on them". I was an insider, as they would show me 'underground' objects and toys.

Discussions with children were loosely structured around the following questions: "What is AIDS?" "How do you get it?" "Do you want to catch it?" "How do you catch it?" and "Can we talk about HIV/AIDS in the classroom?" In relation to these broad questions, children were encouraged to pursue issues that they deemed significant. In ways similar to those reported by Thorne (1993), both boys and girls were strongly invested in constructing themselves in opposition to each other, with many girls describing the boys as immature, irritating and troublesome. Boys also tended to engage with the girls in polarised ways, referring to them as weak and validating their masculinity through the subordination of femininities. However, the polarities were not sustained, with boys and girls positioning themselves within heterosexual cultures, laughing and expressing joy and pleasure whilst talking about dating and kissing. It was boys, however, and 'cool' boys, in particular, who were the objects of greatest female sexual interest.

This study shows that when children were given the opportunity to talk about AIDS, where sex and boyfriends and girlfriends are not off limits (Renold 2005)—issues that are generally considered taboo when in adult company—they were often very keen to do so and showed much emotional engagement. The rich data elicited in the study were, to some extent, because the research was conducted in a sympathetic and non-judgemental way that centred on the children and created opportunities for them to shape and reshape the agenda. Children were aware of the consequences of knowing about sex, and conversations were often punctuated by asking questions and statements such as "Why do you wanna know all this stuff?" "Please, please, please, don't tell the teacher", or "I don't know, I don't know". The interviews were problematic in themselves, with children often negotiating the performance of their sexuality, hiding it and showing awareness of the illicitness of the conversations. By encouraging children to talk about AIDS, sexual desires and concerns in ways that they deemed significant, I acknowledged the child as an expert and as a strategist. Far from giving children rights, the process of doing the research demonstrated how children exercise and negotiate their rights in ways that allow them to hide, display and deny their sexuality. The children were very keen to talk about sexuality. Children felt comfortable to exit as well as talk about sensitive issues that they might not have addressed with parents and teachers. This way of working with young children enables freedom of expression, gives them the confidence to ask, "Why do you want to know all this stuff?" and to refuse to talk and withdraw at their own volition. Anonymity and confidentiality was consistently maintained. Each subject in this study was constantly given the assurance that they were free to express themselves with complete confidentiality.

At KwaDabeka, whilst I sat with children in the classroom in mixed-sex groups, these conversations were restricted by the language. Each group comprised an uneven number of boys and girls. In some groups there was a majority of boys; in others, more girls. In the majority-boys groups, we chatted about soccer and sport (Bhana 2008a). The gendering of groups has effects for what boys and girls can and cannot say. Children, I found, police their knowledge based not only on the embarrassment they felt in relation to the opposite sex but also on the subject matter and the stigma associated with knowing that AIDS is a sex-related disease. Whilst boys and girls did feel embarrassed to say certain things, particularly in relation to sex, the mixed-sex groups allowed for the opportunities for boys and girls to come together, assert their positions and contest each other (Cobbett *et al.* 2013).

The issue of language meant that focus group discussions (with assistance from a translator) were useful at KwaDabeka. Groups of five or six children were withdrawn from the class to a separate room and, with the assistance of a translator, asked questions about the disease. While the process of translation has an impact on the study, the fact that I have some knowledge of isiZulu and the children had some knowledge of English meant there was an element of negotiation between the translator and myself. The scope of the conversations with children varied. The discussion was semi-structured and incorporated the following leading questions: "What is AIDS?" "Who gets AIDS?" and "How do you know who has AIDS?" Within the scope of these broad questions children were encouraged to pursue issues that they deemed significant. As a consequence I rely heavily on the conversations I had with children.

## STRUCTURE OF THE BOOK

Rejecting the passive and marginalised construction of the African child, the chapters in this book show how gender and sexuality permeate and shape children's AIDS-related knowledge. This process is highly complex, as children uphold and break down discourses of childhood innocence whilst simultaneously being enabled and limited by their social contexts. AIDS is produced on the fault lines of social inequalities, but children do come together in expressing knowledge and care for those who are ill. Four of the empirical chapters are devoted to children. Chapters 2, 3, 4 and 5 put children at the centre of this investigation. The data draw extensively from transcribed group discussions, and through the data, I seek to foreground the views and perspectives, the joys, the passions and the plays of power through children's own experiences and voices (Tobin 1997). Chapters 6 and 7 focus on adult narratives of childhood innocence.

### Chapter Outlines

AIDS is made meaningful through a range of discursive processes and children position within these discursive framings as active agents with investments in pleasure, passion and power. In Chapter 2, I bring children from

KwaDabeka and Bullwood together and show the remarkable similarity in the expressions of the disease as AIDS, contagion, kissing, blood, dirt and disease sit alongside AIDS and sex. Children learn from each other as they contest, contribute and reject particular narratives of the disease as they try to fit pieces of the AIDS puzzle together. AIDS stirs up discussion of the 'sexual' routing, and heterosexuality, in particular, is foregrounded as discussion of AIDS and sex provides the moment for boys and girls to discuss various ways in which they come together (and separate) as they talk about heterosexual play (Thorne 1993), kissing and boyfriends and girlfriends (Blaise 2005; Renold 2005; Taylor 2010; Bhana 2013; Robinson 2013). Paradoxically, the chapter illustrates that whilst AIDS is cast within a framework of fear, when it comes to contagion, the connection with sex provides young children with opportunities to explore their sexual and gendered selves.

Chapter 3 focuses on boys and girls at Bullwood. Boys and girls manoeuvre within the discourse of childhood innocence, but they simultaneously manoeuvre the social, economic and cultural context of AIDS in South Africa, and their knowledge is embedded within and contingent on these social processes. This chapter explores the manifestation of stigma in children's responses to the disease. AIDS is constructed as 'catchy' to denote the infectious nature of disease, but complexly intertwines with race, class, age, sexuality and gender. Disease epidemics often breed stigma and people who are infected are often blamed for the disease (Parker & Aggleton 2003; Nattrass 2004). A common response to the AIDS pandemic was this: "Some blacks are getting it." Whilst children distanced themselves from the disease, as the disease of African people, they did so in ways that linked race and class and such constructions are of historical and economic origin, but they also showed a capacity for care and concern for those infected with HIV. The chapter shows the intertwining play of power through a focus on catchy disease, blood, magic, witchdoctors, violence and crime. All come together in the social construction of the disease. The chapter shows how children work on sexual stigma focusing on AIDS as the gay disease, despite its heterosexual spread in South Africa, but they also stigmatise each other for having and possessing sexual knowledge and thus work to police and regulate each other in terms of race, class, age and sexuality.

Chapter 4 turns the focus to KwaDabeka and specifically, the theme of AIDS is rape. The social forces at work in KwaDabeka structure risk for AIDS and such risk complexly shaped by hunger, violence, rape, unemployment, economic distress and cultural notions of male entitlements. AIDS is lodged in this well of misery and economic tragedies over which boys and girls have little control. Power inequalities thus work in different ways in different contexts. The affluence of Bullwood means that it is largely untouched by economic frailties and structural violence (Farmer 2004). Children's understanding of the disease is negotiated within complex social processes involving not only sexual violence and highly unequal gender/age inequalities but also sexual expression. Their sexual expressions, however, are overlaid by fear and are subsumed by a regime of violence, constructing men as chief vectors in the spread of the disease and a source of girls' particular anxieties. As Farmer (2006) has noted, AIDS reveals deeper pathologies of power, and the strikingly unequal social conditions have effects on how boys and girls articulate meanings of the disease, their agency, and their vulnerability and determine who suffers and who is safeguarded.

Chapter 5 returns to boys and girls at Bullwood and KwaDabeka. Here I explore how a declaration of knowing AIDS and not knowing AIDS is rooted in the sexual. The paradox of knowing and not knowing is key to the reproduction of childhood innocence and age relations but also its instability. The chapter considers children's tactical strategies through which the sexual content of AIDS-related knowledge is mediated, negotiated and resisted. Knowing and not knowing are tactical strategies to hide, conceal and reveal sexual knowledge of the disease as children try to constitute intelligible subjects (Davies 1993). Too much sexual knowledge can work against children's status as innocent. In moving within discourses of knowing and not knowing, children move into and out of adult discourses. This chapter approaches children's struggles in weaving in and out of adult discourses within a highly regulatory environment where childhood innocence remains hegemonic. Children hide, deny and silence sex in AIDS-related knowledge enabling childhood to function within familiar relations of power as they contradictorily strengthen and denounce the social fabric of innocence.

Chapter 6 focuses on teachers at Bullwood and KwaDabeka illustrating the deployment of childhood innocence in the sexual constitution of children's AIDS-related knowledge. In doing so, the chapter reveals yet again the paradox of knowing sex and not knowing—from the adult perspective. Dominant discourses silence sexuality and operate within an overall developmental category of thinking about children in ages and stages of development. In managing the paradox, teachers are comfortable linking AIDS to contagion, blood and sexual danger. The dominant features of teaching discourses included the polarization of boys and girls in AIDS education. I argue in this chapter that whilst teachers' constructions are ordered along lines of innocence, there is an implicit assumption that children are, indeed, sexual beings in their framing and warnings about the dangers of having sex.

In Chapter 7, I draw attention to mothers' narratives in the sexual constitution of children's AIDS-related knowledge. The chapter draws attention to the ways in which childhood innocence and child protection is socially constructed and mediated by race and class. Like the teachers in Chapter 6, mothers' combined approach is to shut down sex in AIDS education whilst recognising the need to address sexuality in AIDS education. This paradox is difficult to unravel especially as childhood innocence and child protection dominates their concerns. The chapter identifies the various discursive strategies through which mothers legitimated the sanitization of AIDS-related knowledge including an emphasis on blood and contagion. The chapter also explores the social and discursive contexts through which childhood innocence and child protection are given its force. At KwaDabeka, mothers are vulnerable as material, cultural, symbolic and discursive forces constrain agency as Chapter 4 illustrates about young girls. Childhood innocence, child protection, inequalities, suffering, and power inequalities create similar patterns that reduce women and girls agency and question the social conditions which lead to such vulnerabilities. At Bullwood, the context of privilege produces distancing from and the racialization of AIDS albeit with some level of reflection and reconsideration of hegemonic discourses. Overall, the chapter argues that mothers' approaches generally are antagonistic to sexuality and AIDS education, reproducing dangerous sexuality and child protection. However, beyond these negative framings are the possibilities of working with mothers to reflect on childhood innocence, child protection and distancing mechanisms in operation at Bullwood.

The final chapter, Chapter 8, identifies some of the key findings that expand upon the central claims made regarding the ways in which children's AIDS-related sexual knowledge is expressed, negotiated, resisted and regulated. Children's understanding of AIDS, both contests and promotes childhood innocence whilst simultaneously the effect of material, cultural, symbolic and discursive forces which creates greater vulnerability for girls. My intention in the conclusion is not to provide a step-by-step guide to effective sexuality education and AIDS education. The main argument I make is that adults need to unravel the paradox of childhood innocence, sexuality and AIDS education and to start early in addressing children as social, sexual and gendered beings. Childhood innocence is a major argument used for precluding sexuality in AIDS education because children are deemed to be too young to know and lacking the maturity to deal with the sexual matters of life. When children's voices are put at the centre, the paradox begins to unravel, summoning a rethinking of the silences that continually make children vulnerable. In rethinking sexuality and AIDS education researchers need to work with what children consider as relevant and we need to begin where children are at (Aggleton & Campbell 2000; Allen 2011). The focus on adult narratives combined with children's testimonies provides rich data to address and unravel the AIDS paradox whilst paying attention to the deeper pathologies of power. Any policy development must take heed of children's actual realities and the operation of power, which are considered in the rest of the book.

## NOTES

1  Pseudonyms are used throughout text.
2  In this book I use the term *AIDS*. AIDS is caused by HIV, human immunodeficiency virus. HIV destroys the body's ability to fight off infection, which could lead to death. My decision to use the terms *AIDS*, *AIDS related* and *AIDS education* is to improve the book's readability (see UNAIDS Terminology Guidelines, 2011).

3 Under the apartheid system of segregation (1948–1994), the population of South Africa was classified according to four racial categories: African, white, Indian (referring to family origins from any part of the Indian sub-continent) and 'coloured' (referring to mixed or diverse racial origins). While there is no longer a legislated system of racial classification, nor is race stable, the apartheid-defined racial terms continue to be used both colloquially and formally. In this study, I have used the term *African* instead of *black*. This was intentional and speaks to a decision not to reinforce the dehumanising social structures and labels of apartheid. While many South Africans self-identify as black, this descriptor can produce homogeneity because the majority who live in KwaDabeka are poor and African. It is hoped that 'African' here speaks to the need for empowering identity markers that acknowledge the structural, economic and racial inequalities in South Africa (see Bhana, 2014).

## REFERENCES

Aggleton, P. & Campbell, C. (2000), 'Working with young people – towards an agenda for sexual health', *Sexual and Relationship Therapy*, 15(3): 283-296.

Alanen, L. (1997) 'The politics of growing up', Paper presented to the 'Children 5–16: Growing Into The 21st Century' Conference, Keele University. 17 March.

Alderson, P. (2007) 'Competent Children? Minors' Consent to Health Care Treatment and Research'. *Social Science and Medicine*, 65: 2272–2283.

Allen, L. (2011) *Young People and Sexuality Education: Rethinking Key Debates*. New York: Palgrave Macmillan.

Barbarin, O. A. & Richter, L. (2001) *Mandela's Children*. New York: Routledge.

Bhana, D. (2007) 'The Price of Innocence: Teachers, Gender, Childhood Sexuality, HIV and AIDS in Early Schooling'. *International Journal of Inclusive Education*, 11(4): 431–444.

Bhana, D. (2008a) 'Beyond Stigma? Young Children's Responses to HIV and AIDS'. *Culture, Health & Sexuality*, 10(7): 725–738.

Bhana, D. (2008b) ' "Six Packs and Big Muscles, and Stuff Like That" Primary School-Aged South African Boys Black and White, on Sport'. *British Journal of Sociology of Education*, 29(1): 3–14.

Bhana, D. (2012) ' "Girls Are not Free" in and out of the South African School'. *International Journal of Educational Development*, 32(2): 352–358.

Bhana, D. (2013) 'Kiss and Tell: Boys, Girls and Sexualities in the Early Years'. *Agenda*, 27(3): 57–66.

Bhana, D. (2014) *Under Pressure: The Regulation of Sexualities in South African Secondary Schools*. Braamfontein: Mathoko's Books.

Bhana, D. & Farook Brixen, F. (with MacNaughton, G. & Zimmerman, R.) (2006) *Children, HIV/AIDS and Gender: A Summary Review*. Working paper 39. The Hague: Bernard van-Leer Foundation.

Bhana, D. & Singh, S. (2012) 'Gender, Sexuality and HIV and AIDS Education in South Africa'. *The Impact of HIV/AIDS on Education Worldwide*, 18: 213–230.

Blaise, M. (2005) 'A Feminist Poststructuralist Study of Children "Doing" Gender in an Urban Kindergarten Classroom'. *Early Childhood Research Quarterly*, 20(1): 85–108.

Bray, R., Gooskens, I., Kahn, L., Moses, S. & Seekings, J. (2010) *Growing Up in the New South Africa: Childhood and Adolescence in the New South Africa*. Cape Town: Human Sciences, Research Council Press.

Burman, S. B. & Reynolds, P. (1986) (eds) *Growing Up in a Divided Society: The Contexts of Childhood in South Africa*. Johannesburg: Raven Press.

Butler, J. (1990) *Gender Trouble: Feminism and the Subversion of Identity*. New York: Routledge.

Clark, J. (2014) 'Sexualisation and the Discursive Figure of the Child'. *Sociological Studies of Children and Youth*, 18: 173–197.

Cobbett, M., McLaughlin, C. & Kiragu, S. (2013) 'Creating "Participatory Spaces": Involving Children in Planning Sex Education Lessons in Kenya, Ghana and Swaziland'. *Sex Education*, 13(1): 70–83.

Corrêa, S., Petchesky, R. & Parker, R. (2008) *Sexuality, Health and Human Rights*. London: Routledge.

Davies, B. (1993) *Shards of Glass: Children Reading and Writing Beyond Gendered Identities*. St. Leonards, NSW: Allen and Unwin.

Department of Education. (1998) *National Norms and Standards*. Pretoria: Department of Education.

Department of Education. (2006) *Amended National Norms and Standards for School Funding*. Pretoria: Department of Education.

Egan, R.D. (2013) *Becoming Sexual: A Critical Appraisal of the Sexualization of Girls*. Oxford: Polity Press.

Egan, R.D. & Hawkes, G. (2009) 'The Problem With Protection: Or, Why We Need to Move Towards Recognition and the Sexual Agency of Children'. *Continuum: Journal of Media & Cultural Studies*, 23(3): 389–400.

Epstein, D. & Johnson, R. (1998) *Schooling Sexualities*. Buckingham: Open University Press.

Farmer, P. (2004) 'An Anthropology of Structural Violence 1'. *Current Anthropology*, 45(3): 305–325.

Farmer, P. (2006) *AIDS and Accusation: Haiti and the Geography of Blame*. Berkeley: University of California Press.

Frosh, S., Phoenix, A. & Pattman, R. (2002) *Young Masculinities: Understanding Boys in Contemporary Society*. London: Palgrave.

Foucault, M. (1977) *Discipline and Punish*: New York: Pantheon.

Foucault, M. (1980) *Power/Knowledge: Selected Interviews and Other Writings 1972–1977*. Hemel Hempstead: Harvester.

HSRC (Human Sciences Research Council). (2005) *South African National HIV Prevalence, HIV Incidence, Behaviour and Communication Survey, 2005*. Cape Town: HSRC Press.

Ingraham, C. (1996) 'The Heterosexual Imaginary: Feminist Sociology and Theories of Gender', in S. Seidman (ed) *Queer Theory/Sociology* (pp. 168–193). Cambridge, MA: Blackwell.

Jackson, S. & Scott, S. (2010) *Theorizing Sexuality*. Maidenhead: McGraw-Hill-Open University Press.

James, A., Jenks, C. & Prout, A. (1998) *Theorising Childhood*. Cambridge: Polity Press.

Galtung, J. (1969) Violence, Peace and Peace Research. *Journal of Peace Research*, 6: 167–191.

Jones, S. (1993) *Assaulting Childhood: Children's Experiences of Migrancy and Hostel Life in South Africa*. Johannesburg: Witwatersrand University Press.

Kane, E.W. (2013) *Rethinking Gender and Sexuality in Childhood*. New York: Bloomsbury.

Karim, Q.A., Kharsany, A.B.M., Leask, K., Ntombela, F., Humphries, H., Frohlich, J.A., Samsunder, N., Grobler, A., Dellar, R. & Karim, S.S.A. (2014) 'Prevalence of HIV, HSV-2 and Pregnancy Among High School Students in Rural KwaZulu-Natal, South Africa: A Bio-Behavioural Cross-Sectional Survey'. *Epidemiology*, 90(8): 620–627.

Kincaid, J.R. (1998) *Erotic Innocence: The Culture of Child Molesting*. Durham, NC: Duke University Press.

Kippax, S., Stephenson, N., Parker, R. G. & Aggleton, P. (2013) 'Between Individual Agency and Structure in HIV Prevention: Understanding the Middle Ground of Social Practice'. *American Journal of Public Health*, 103(8): 1367–1375.

MacNaughton, G. (2000) *Rethinking Gender in Early Childhood Education*. London: Paul Chapman.

Mayall, B. (2002) *Towards a Sociology for Childhood: Thinking From Children's Lives*. Buckingham: Open University Press.

Miedema, E., Maxwell, C. & Aggleton, P. (2015) 'The Unfinished Nature of Rights Informed HIV- and AIDS-Related Education: An Analysis of Three School-Based Initiatives'. *Sex Education: Sexuality, Society and Learning*, 15(1): 78–92.

Morrell, R., Epstein, D., Unterhalter, E., Bhana, D. & Moletsane, R. (2009) *Towards Gender Equality? South African Schools During the HIV/AIDS Epidemic*. Pietermaritzburg: University of KwaZulu-Natal Press.

Nattrass, N. (2004) *The Moral Economy of AIDS in South Africa*. Cambridge: Cambridge University Press.

Parker, R (2001). "Sexuality, Culture, and Power in HIV/AIDS Research". *Annual Review of Anthropology* 30: 163–179.

Parker, R. (2009) 'Sexuality, Culture and Society: Shifting Paradigms in Sexuality Research'. *Culture, Health & Sexuality: An International Journal for Research, Intervention and Care*, 11(3): 251–266.

Parker, R. & Aggleton, P. (2003) 'HIV and AIDS-Related Stigma and Discrimination: A Conceptual Framework and Implications for Action'. *Social science & Medicine*, 57(1): 13–24.

Parsons, R. (2012) *Growing Up With HIV in Zimbabwe. One Day This Will Be Over*. Harare: James Currey, Weaver Press.

Ramphele, M. (2002) *Steering by the Stars: Being Young in South Africa*. Cape Town: Tafelberg.

Renold, E. (2005) *Girls, Boys and Junior Sexualities: Exploring Children's Gender and Sexual Relations in the Primary School*. London: Routledge Falmer.

Reynolds, P. (1989) *Childhood in Crossroads: Cognition and society in South Africa*. Cape Town: David Phillip Grand Rapids.

Robinson, K. (2013) *Innocence, Knowledge and the Construction of Childhood: The Contradictory Nature of Sexuality and Censorship in Children's Contemporary Lives*. New York: Routledge.

Save the Children. (2007) *Tell Me More! Children's Rights and Sexuality in the Context of HIV/AIDS in Africa*. Sweden: RFSU.

Sedgwick, E. K. (1990) *The Epistemology of the Closet*. Berkeley: University of California Press.

Shisana, O., Rehle, T., Simbayi, L.C., Zuma, K., Jooste, S. & Zungu, N. (2014) *South African National HIV Prevalence, Incidence and Behaviour Survey, 2012*. Cape Town: HSRC Press.

Silin, J. (1995) *Sex, Death and the Education of Children: Our Passion for Ignorance in the Age of AIDS*. New York: Teachers College Press.

Statistics South Africa (2014) *Mid-Year Population Estimates*. Pretoria: Statistics South Africa.

Taylor, Y. (ed) (2010) *Classed Intersections: Space, Selves, Knowledges*. Aldershot: Ashgate.

Therborn, G. (2013) *The Killing Fields of Inequality*. Cambridge: Polity Press.

Thorne, B. (1993) *Gender Play: Girls and Boys in School*. Brunswick: Rutgers University Press.

Tobin, J. (1997) 'The Missing Discourse of Pleasure and Desire', in J. Tobin (ed) *Making a Place for Pleasure in Early Childhood Education* (pp. 1–37). New Haven, CT: Yale University Press.

UNAIDS (2011) *Terminology Guidelines*. Geneva: UNAIDS.

UNESCO (United Nations Educational, Scientific and Cultural Organization). (2009) *International Technical Guidance on Sexuality Education: An Evidence-informed Approach for Schools, Teachers and Health Educators, Vol 1—Rationale for sexuality Education.* Paris: UNESCO.

Weeks, J. (1986) *Sexuality.* London: Routledge.

Weeks, J. (2000) *Making Sexual History.* Cambridge: Polity Press.

Wood, L & Rolleri, L. A. (2014) 'Designing an Effective Sexuality Education Control Themselves': Teachers' Beliefs and Attitudes Towards Young People's Sexual and Curriculum for Schools: Lessons Gleaned From the South(ern) African Literature'. *Sex Education: Sexuality, Society and Learning*, 14(5): 525–542.

# 2 AIDS, Sex and Disease
## How Much Do Boys and Girls Know?

| | |
|---|---|
| Daniel: | I heard something. I heard someone has AIDS . . . He kissed that person on the lips and then got AIDS . . . it will go into you and you will get it. . . |
| Mitchell: | No, you get it by having sex. . . [laughs and giggles]. When people are making. . . [laughing] . . . When people [laughing in the background] when people are making out and then they kiss [Group discussion at *Bullwood*] |
| Sanelisiwe(g): | The boys go and sleep with the girls and they get AIDS. |

—Conversation at KwaDabeka

How do boys and girls at KwaDabeka and Bullwood, interpret, shape and negotiate their knowledge of disease. This chapter explores the nuanced ways in which AIDS is conceptualised as it foregrounds boys and girls investment in sexuality. The ways in which children connect AIDS, sex and gender is not simple. Children do link disease to sex as the earlier quotes suggest, but children's AIDS-related knowledge is messy, and their knowledge of sex is also linked to contagion and kissing (Bhana & Epstein 2007). Talk about sex and disease appears suddenly, unpredictably and momentarily, because children contest and challenge each other as they enact, display and express gender and sexuality. It was impossible to talk about the disease without children actively linking sexual knowledge of the disease within heterosexual cultures and practices and through which gender relations of power were expressed. The sexual connection with the disease was accompanied by laughter and giggles, suggesting both children's pleasure in the articulation of sexuality and the shame and embarrassment that governs and polices, as children police their knowledge of sexuality. In the first section of this chapter, I examine the ways in which boys and girls connect AIDS with sex and sexuality, transgressing discourses of childhood innocence, not only because they express pleasure in contesting each other but also because they come together through heterosexual activities such as play, kissing and sexual cultures involving boyfriends of girlfriends. Whilst AIDS is cast within a framework of contagion, its intimate connection with sex provided young children with opportunities to explore, express and negotiate their sexual and gendered selves. In the second part of this chapter I focus on sexual danger and the ways in which gender binaries are created through the 'bad man' discourse, which sees male power pitted against innocent girls. The overall context of male power and male violence is imbricated in their understanding of AIDS, rape and male power. Chapter 4 gives special attention to the construction of "AIDS is rape" at KwaDabeka.

## AIDS IS SEX/GENDER

When sex features in young children's discussion of the route of HIV transmission, it is important to recognise that such revelations occur in the context in which children's right to sexual information is often restricted and considered inappropriate and problematic (Robinson 2005). This does not mean that children's realities sit comfortably with adult wishes about innocence because Amy's response to the question of how to get AIDS involves attempts to describe sex and sexual activity.

## Bullwood

| | |
|---|---|
| Amy: | Okay . . . [laughing] when you want to have a baby [laughing] when you have a baby, you have sex and you kiss and they like to put their tongues inside each other's mouth . . . yuck . . . |
| Arend: | That's smooching. |
| Amy: | No that's kissing. . . . |
| Jason: | All people do that. . . . |
| Annie: | I won't say anything about that. |
| Jennifer: | Okay, . . . it's when . . . people when people like each other and they like do it and kiss [laughing]. |
| Sara: | My mum said that, I asked her about it. She said that there's a special kind of relationship between a man and a woman. The kind . . . [laughing] . . . It's like when a man . . . I don't know. I don't know. |
| Josina: | There's a special kind of relationship between a man and a woman. *Ja.* |
| Tash: | And then when . . . when . . . I don't know. Something happens and then the man must have AIDS and he can pass it on to the woman . . . onto that person between the relationship. I don't know how. |

Children's language of sex and AIDS is embedded within an environment where laughter is common, especially as sex is seen as something shameful for young children. But children in this study also demonstrate sexual curiosity with the confidence to engage in conversations about sexuality and to make clear this knowledge in the route of HIV transmission. Ambivalent, they are also reluctant to pursue a conversation around the sexual route of transmission where they know that their knowledge of sex is taboo for young seven- and eight-year-old children. Annie, unlike Amy, says, "I won't say anything about that". Recent work has established the ambivalence that young children demonstrate in the performance of sexuality distancing as an age-appropriate endeavour that not only gives meaning to innocence but also invests in sexuality by asserting their sexual selves through conversations about boyfriends and love letters and by establishing heterosexual desirability (Blaise 2010; Robinson 2013). In explaining sex and AIDS, Amy tries to make the connection among reproduction, sex and sexual activity, such as kissing, with the focus on the tongue—which generates for her as a child a level of disgust. Whilst these revelations are in contrast to adult assumptions about childhood innocence, Amy, too, as an eight-year-old, depicts sexual activity, and particularly the "tongues inside each other's mouth", with the expression "yuck" to symbolise sexual activity as disgusting, particularly from a child's standpoint where such activity is not only disallowed but considered inappropriate to childhood. Children are thus active makers of sexuality whilst resisting and locking into discourses of innocence. The repulsion at kissing is a justifiable response particularly considering the risks involved in projecting an overt sexuality at age eight. Not only did the children set the sexual agenda as far as their knowledge of AIDS is concerned, but they also showed a great deal of sophistication in linking sex, multiple partners and AIDS, as the conversation with Johan and Steven at Bullwood illustrates:

> Johan: If you go around with other girls like sleep around . . . Like it goes the different way. The other easier way is, when someone has AIDS and you got a sore like say over here and say someone has a sore like here and say you swing your arm and touch the blood then you get AIDS . . . The other way is like when you have sex, you know, when you have sex like with other people, they're not your own wife.
>
> DB: Which other people?
>
> Johan: Like say Steven is my wife, and I go with other people then I would [get] AIDS. Just say someone is here and someone is here and this one is my wife and this one is not [pointing], I will go out with this one. I will probably get AIDS. Then you probably fall in love and then you'll have sex and then you probably get AIDS.
>
> Steven: But there is one question, but I don't know how you get it?
>
> Johan: I don't know. I got to bring my book to school. I got a book all about sex.
>
> DB: Who gave that book to you?
>
> Johan: My mum . . . it says like, when you like married and two of you really like each other, then they go around and have sex.

Clearly, Johan's knowledge of the disease is enabled by the home context where his mother (unlike most) had provided him with access to a book about relationships and sex. He tries to explain that having many sexual partners and sex outside of marriage creates vulnerability to disease. This conversation, like the next one at Bullwood, was intricately intertwined with contagion—though sex and disease brought different kinds of emotional responses. The sexual transmission brought pleasure and fun to the fore as boys and girls inserted into heterosexual cultures and disease; germs brought death and illness together.

In the following transcript the children talked about the dangers of coming into contact with the blood of people infected with HIV:

> Megan:  Sometimes you get a cut and then you touch their blood and you can get AIDS from that 'cause that blood has germs and other sicknesses in it. All that germs goes into your blood and you touch it and you get AIDS.
>
> Sarah:  Like when you have blood and you have AIDS and then your friend touches and she forgot that you have AIDS then she also gets it from you.

Both Sarah and Megan were alert to the connection between AIDS and blood, but their knowledge of the disease was underscored by the fear of contagion and their vulnerability to disease, so the tone of the conversation was very serious. But the seriousness and the fear were quickly defused when Candice referred to sex:

> Candice:  . . . [I]f you sleep with a boy . . . [laughing] and you sleep together and then you get AIDS . . . [laughing]
>
> DB:  What's sleep?
>
> Candice:  They sleep . . . [laughing]
>
> DB:  Sleep?
>
> Donovan:  No like if a boy is sleeping and a girl is sleeping with him together. Sleeping together.
>
> DB:  I thought you get AIDS from blood.
>
> Sarah:  Like when you sleep together . . . [laughing]
>
> Megan:  Yes, you sleep together, I mean the boy and girl they sleep together and you have AIDS and the boy does not wear a condom, like that.
>
> Sarah:  Or you could say, that if you are a man and you have AIDS and you don't wear a condom then that girl would get AIDS and she would need to go to the hospital.
>
> DB:  What's a condom?
>
> Sarah:  Condom?
>
> DB:  Yes. What is that?

Kate:      It's like a word that you use when you don't want to have a baby.

Donovan:  No it's not a word. It looks like a balloon and its white and then they do something and the boy puts it on. [laughing]

Children's understanding of AIDS is closely related to their knowledge of sexual behaviour and prevention, as suggested by the discussion about the condom. Strikingly, the shift in conversation from blood to sex was also an emotional shift from the fear, anxiety and vulnerability associated with the potent symbols of blood and AIDS, to embarrassment, laughter, giggles and pleasure as heterosexuality was expressed. In other words, through their constructions of AIDS the children were exploring their own positions in a heterosexual society. Interestingly, once Candice destroyed the myth of innocence, Sarah and Megan were keen to pursue the conversation about sleeping together without drawing on the previous conversation about infection and blood and its resonance with fear. Rather, the conversation became a means for the children to articulate their sexual desires and knowledge.

## Bullwood

Rita:     I dumped Zane.

DB:      How do you get dumped?

Rita:     You just say, "I don't want to be friends anymore". Every time Zane comes around and touches me, sometimes he does it, but sometimes I am the one who goes and touches him.

DB:      So when do you do that?

Rita:     Like when we play "tag" and try and run away.

Boyfriends, dumping, touching and playing tag are routine and highly expected forms of sexualised routines for seven- and eight-year-olds—from their point of view. The discussion about AIDS moves to boyfriends and Rita talks about dumping Zane, to touching Zane (as he also does) to playing tag. As other research has shown tag is gendered and sexualised (Thorne 1993)—involving sexualised running on the school playgrounds whilst violating childhood innocence and bringing boys and girls together.

The children's knowledge of AIDS and its close association with sex and sexuality were enabled through the support of the group as the myth of innocence was shattered. That the conversation moved from blood to sex with the support of the group meant that each child was giving another a point of access to a (hetero)sexual (and gendered) discourse as the conversation shifted from the dangers of AIDS infection through contact with infected blood to sex. Within this complex matrix, heterosexual desirability was projected and validated in the group support of one other. The children took delight and pleasure in talking about sex and in this way they were learning to become part of a sexual culture where at any point in the conversation sex talk and condoms were foregrounded. The discussion about the condom did not simply destroy the myth of childhood innocence but also provided the children with the knowledge that condoms provide protection against HIV and pregnancy.

## KwaDabeka

> Prince:   I'm going to get married.
> DB:       Why?
> Lindo:    My wife can make salad for me.
> Prince:   Girls give us surprises.
> DB:       Surprises?
> Prince:   . . . [H]aving a date.
> DB:       What is a "date"?
> Prince:   A date is like going to a restaurant and having some food . . . Like give the girl a rose and maybe say like . . . will you marry me . . . when you have a ring.

The preceding discussion at KwaDabeka arose when children talked about the sexual transmission of the disease. Heterosexual love is ever present and is embedded within imagined heterosexual futures, idealisation of marriage and heterosexual activities involving dates and heterosexual practices that cement relationships—the rose and the ring in this case is the hard evidence of heterosexual masculinity.

> Winnie:   The other day Prince when he was with us, me and Thuli and Luyanda and Lindo . . . I said, "Prince, can you please borrow us your book, we want to write?" It was a spare book . . . he said, "Let me write the message" . . . then we saw the message in the book saying, "I love you, I love you", then we saw that and Prince said, "Let me write a letter to both of you" and then he writes, "I love you Thuli" and "Winnie . . . you are sexy" . . . and then I said, "We don't love you because you're ugly . . . you are like a shorty *makoti* [Zulu bride]!"

Here Winnie shows how masculinity, sexuality and power are connected in the heterosexual bind. Prince is able to assert his heterosexuality by declaring his love for Thuli, and the use of the word *sexy* serves as a confirmation of boys' heterosexual masculinity. The love letter serves to instantiate heterosexual practice and to claim power, albeit only temporarily because Winnie cast Prince as ugly and the love is not reciprocated. In this conversation with Winnie there was a great deal of laughter and enjoyment as Winnie narrated the story about Prince. I asked her what *sexy* meant:

Winnie:    When you are beautiful and wearing short things and then say you are so beautiful and sexy and you are going like this . . . [sways her hips].

Winnie's power and agency are produced through the love letter contradicting the discourse of childhood innocence whilst being seduced into fun, laughter and pleasure through the hard copy of the heterosexual male gaze. Even though Winnie protests against Prince's declaration of sexiness and love, her definition of being sexy revolves around heterosexual desirability, wearing short things and being beautiful as she sways her hips. This discussion functions as an investment into heterosexual femininity and desirability because it exceeds the normative understanding of childhood innocence.

Laughter as I have argued is an important area in understanding the projection of heterosexual desire amongst young boys and girls (Allen 2014). These conversations, for example, were loaded with giggles, smiles and laughter as talk about sex invoked the senses in pleasurable ways. In addition, the place of play is a defining feature of children's emerging sexual cultures (Thorne 1993). In this study, the game of kiss and catch was a powerful means through which sexuality was forged in the open spaces of the school ground. Children spoke pleasurably about boyfriends and girlfriends and about kissing and dating and talked at length about kiss-kiss-chase games, which functioned not only to reproduce their sexual identities but also to break down gender boundaries.

## KwaDabeka

Similarly at KwaDabeka, discussions show how prominently sexual matters feature in children's AIDS-related knowledge:

DB:            How exactly is AIDS spread?
Mlondi (b):    By kissing [giggles].
Wendy:         They're naughty [laughs]. They take off their clothes and have sex.
DB:            What's that?
Wendy:         It's when you are going to make a child.
Wendy:         By playing with boys.
Nosiphu (g):   Sleeping with him. People get naughty in bed [laughs].
Scelo (b):     By not wearing a condom.

In these discussions, children connect AIDS with sex and sexual behaviour and, in doing so, transgress the myths of sexual innocence. Enabled by support from their peers, and accompanied by laughter, these children were able to talk about sex within the wider constraints of sexual taboos and in ways that enable them to insert themselves into a sexual culture. Laughter acquires a symbolic significance in this context. Not only does it allow for the validation and support of childhood sexual cultures; it also allows them to speak of transgression. Their knowledge about condoms does not simply break the myth of childhood innocence but also provides the young children with an awareness of the safety that the condom is supposed to provide against AIDS. But while children are asserting their right to know sexually and enjoy the conversation, judgement is also passed on sex as "naughty". The significance of sex as "naughty" highlights the ways in which young children take the meaning of sex—as both pleasurable (using the logic of laughter) and naughty (adopting an adult stance). In other words, young children express sexuality but also adopt adult stances on the matter, distancing and rejecting child sex. In this way, they adjust and accommodate their right to know sexually.

## AIDS IS SEX, GENDER AND DANGER

Children's knowledge of AIDS is strongly influenced by their experiences and their localities. Not only is South African AIDS a national emergency but there is also a considerable gender disparity in the rates of infection, with women and girls being most vulnerable to infection (Shisana et al. 2014). Young South African children are not oblivious to these gendered issues; they are very responsive to their social environments where sexual violence is acute.

### Bullwood

| | |
|---|---|
| Brenda: | It's mostly the boys that spread AIDS 'cause they want the girls and stuff. |
| Beatrice: | Sometimes it's girls . . . |
| Brenda: | No, it's boys who rape the girls . . . |
| DB: | What's rape? |
| Mitchell: | You stop a girl and you force her to have sex with you. |
| DB: | Who's doing this? |
| Mitchell: | Boys that break into houses and that kind of stuff. |

AIDS, rape and the victimisation of girls occur in a context where tales of violence and sexual violence have featured prominently in South African society (with African boys and young men being constructed as the perpetrators). Children's responses to AIDS show the intimate connections between sex and gender, where both boys and girls have an acute sense of understanding gender inequalities and sexual violence. When Brenda responds to Beatrice's claim that girls also contribute to AIDS, she disputes this and is supported by Mitchell. Brenda's knowledge of women's vulnerability (and resilience) draws from a true story of a white South African woman Alison (Thamm 2002), who refused to become a victim of rape. Despite being raped, stabbed and having her throat slit and left for dead near the city of Port Elizabeth in the Eastern Cape Province of South Africa, she defied death and has become an icon in South Africa as a woman who conquered sexual violence:

> Brenda:   I read this book. My mum read this book. It's called *I Have Life*. It's about like a million or 500 books that are being sold. This one girl told her that she actually survived. These two men opened her stomach until all the outsides were out, the insides were out. Around her neck, here, and all over her tummy, they ripped her insides to the outside. And they were showing it, not when it was open, when they stitched it about how they stitched it. And her face is on the front of the book and she's like the prettiest girl. She is so beautiful and has long hair and she said I have life 'cause her mother told her you have life. She thought of what her mother said that you can never give up. The mother said that she must go and have a life and try and do something. They even show you the knife that they used to cut her open.

Brenda's contestation of Beatrice's version of girls in the spread of AIDS thus draws from her graphic description of sexual and physical violence as recounted from the true story of Alison. The ways in which gender inequalities operate to reinforce prevailing power structures, a rampant heterosexual masculinity which leads to unsafe and violent sexual relations and the impact of these gendered and sexual dynamics in the rates of infection are now well documented in South Africa (Hunter 2005). Brenda's knowledge draws from her social context, her engagement with her mother through reading and the conversation about AIDS provides a platform through which she asserts her gendered and sexual knowledge, arguing her point with vivid descriptions of violence and resilience.

At Bullwood, working-class African girls who chatted with me during the break as we sat on the playground were hesitant to speak about AIDS and sex when in the group. This suggests that the African girls' knowledge of sexuality is highly policed by peers, and the relative freedom offered to them during the interviews on the playground asserted their right to be heard. The two girls in the conversation that follows were African working-class girls whose mothers were domestic workers in Bullwood. Their fees are subsidised by independent newspapers, and they are highly aware that, because of their particular class location, they would not have been able to secure a place at the school without the subsidy. In the conversations that follow it must be noted that the tension between danger and pleasure is very powerful.

Sexuality is simultaneously a field of restriction, repression and danger as well as a domain of pleasure and agency through which gender is constructed. Sexuality is nuanced by other social differences so different cultural and social backgrounds make available not only different versions of masculinity and femininity but different versions of sexuality (Epstein & Johnson 1998). The children, in their conversation, pick up on the danger that sexuality represents to girls and the ways in which fear of AIDS polices and regulates sexuality. The ways in which girls from a working-class context make meaning of their sexuality will be contextually specific (Hey 1997). Social class makes available not only different versions of masculinity and femininity but different versions of sexuality:

| | |
|---|---|
| Gugu: | AIDS is something like when you're sick, and like people don't hear about the things. If you have a sore and then a person touches your blood than you also get AIDS from them. Maybe when that person is sick then she has AIDS. Then when you touch the blood then you gonna get sick like them. |
| Thobeka: | Yes. I have heard that if someone touches you, but don't touch your blood but they touch your skin you won't get AIDS. |
| DB: | How would you say, okay, that a person's got AIDS? |
| Gugu: | They have to go and test. |
| DB: | How do you test? |
| Thobeka: | They have to, um, um, I don't know. They put an injection on you and then they have to test the blood or something like that. I don't know. |
| Gugu: | When they go to test you they . . . like, there is something they put on you then see how much blood you have with AIDS. It's like a special ruler thing. |
| DB: | What does it do? |
| Thobeka: | It tests your blood. |

Gugu and Thobeka showed a great deal more sophistication in their knowledge of AIDS and the relationship between AIDS, illness, sores and blood than did girls like Sarah and Megan. This was the easy part for the girls since the association with sex remained absent. However, when asked what AIDS meant they immediately offered a response through laughter, giggling and smiles:

| | |
|---|---|
| DB: | What does AIDS mean? |
| Thobeka: | Don't even speak about it. [laughing and giggling] |
| Gugu: | AIDS means when you have boy and have sex and both of you don't wear a condom. [giggling] |
| DB: | How do you know so much? |
| Gugu: | I heard it on TV that if you don't wear it, then if that person has AIDS and then you got infected. |

| | |
|---|---|
| Thobeka: | If you don't wear it then you'll get AIDS from him or her. [laughing] |
| DB: | You can get AIDS from boys and girls? |
| Gugu: | Boys! |
| DB: | Boys. Why, Thobeka? |
| Gugu: | Definitely boys. |
| DB: | Why? |
| Thobeka: | Maybe they have, like, have other girlfriends and they have AIDS and they sleep together and then now he has it, yes? |
| Gugu: | If you have got one partner and you and they go to another girl they both got AIDS. |
| DB: | And are boys doing this? |
| Gugu: | Yes. They try to rape the girls. |
| DB: | They try to rape the girls? |
| Thobeka: | Yes. My aunt says that if the girl, you know, like when you finish bathing and you have no clothes on, a boy would obviously see you and take you and sleep with you then you'll get AIDS. Let's say the door is open in the kitchen and your rooms also opened and you're showering and then when you come out and then behind you the boy takes you and then he rapes you and then you get AIDS and then you get a baby and you die. |
| Gugu: | My mum said I mustn't play on my own and, um, play by my house, 'cause if a person comes and chases me then they will rape me, and then I'll get AIDS. |
| DB: | What is rape? |
| Thobeka: | I don't know. When you set a girl up. |
| Gugu: | *Ja*, when you set a girl up. Like say gonna meet her somewhere at the corner there and you hide and you attack her. |
| DB: | You attack her? How do you know that? |
| Thobeka: | My aunt told me that. |
| DB: | So what is rape? |
| Gugu: | I'm so scared to say. |
| DB: | Don't be afraid. Say it quietly. |
| Thobeka: | I know what it is. |
| Gugu: | Sex, sex. [laughing] |
| Thobeka: | When you sleep with a girl, when a boy puts his penis into the girls' vagina. [laughing] |
| DB: | How do you know that? |
| Gugu: | We saw it on the TV. And you know *loveLife*? |
| Thobeka: | My cousin had this book and I have seen it there was a girl and the boy came inside and after that they sleep together. |

Children know a great deal about gender and sexuality, but this does not mean that they all know the same things (Epstein *et al.* 2003). Childhood sexuality must be seen in relation to the social and material context surrounding the institution of heterosexuality. The context of many children in South Africa is characterised by massive economic and social disadvantage, sexual violence and the HIV epidemic. Their knowledge of AIDS and their articulation of gender and sexuality can only occur through their particular circumstances. Young children exhibit their sexuality in ways that reflect their own circumstances. African working-class girls are much more vulnerable to rape and the risk of HIV infection, because they live in a crucible of poverty, violence and social distress.

Thobeka and Gugu showed a great deal of knowledge about personal and sexual issues and television programmes and magazines such as *loveLife* (a magazine supporting safe sex in South Africa) provide a platform for sharing and debating such knowledge. Their social, material and cultural world was really significant to their understanding of AIDS, sex and sexuality. Whilst they could see the pleasurable side of sex and showed a great deal of emotion in this regard, their pleasure was overlaid by the material and social circumstances in South Africa which make African working-class women vulnerable to rape and abuse. The emergent sexuality and agency of African, working-class girls is constrained by their knowledge of what happens to girls: rape, pregnancy, AIDS and death. Given the legacies of apartheid, the history of inequalities, a violent and a highly patriarchal system of government and the calamitous socio-economic conditions which continue to emasculate African men, it is little surprise that the girls construct their femininities and sexualities by drawing on discourses of fear of men, rape and AIDS (Hunter 2005). Gugu's and Thobeka's responses demonstrate the intimate links between sexuality, culture, material and social forces and their own positioning as children with sexual knowledge. For these girls, sexuality is framed by, and overlaid with, fear. However, the broader discourses about men and the danger that they represent also inhabit the positions that many middle-class white girls adopt:

> Estelle:   I watched a movie about a little girl and her mum and dad and her sister. Her mum said lets go the shops and they went to the shops and the girl got lost.
> DB:   What happened to the girl?
> Estelle:   The girl went into the shops and her mum was waiting for her in the car. There were two men; they caught the little girl in the back . . . there's bad men, there's lots of bad men around and they could kill you 'cause the men are very vicious and strong. I think that it is normally the men who do that.

The polarisation of gendered identities occurs within the bad men discourse, which sees masculine strength, violence and aggression pitted against innocent girls. Estelle's recollection of the movie scene is not isolated. Her fear is real. Tales of violence and sexual violence have featured prominently in

South African society (with African boys and young men being constructed as the perpetrators). However, in South Africa it is more likely that African girls will be victims of African male violence. Violence and sexual violence among young African men in South Africa are acute (Hunter 2005). African men have been particularly problematised in the context of the HIV epidemic, with campaigns and literature addressing them, especially, as people with multiple partners who engage in forms of sexual harassment and violence.

## CONCLUSION

The image of the child as innocent and too young to understand abstract issues relating to disease is not one which stands up to scrutiny when children are given the opportunity and space to talk about AIDS, as shown in this chapter. The children in this study proved themselves to be curious, knowledgeable and capable of thoughtful reflection, and their responses, questions and struggles in making sense of the disease are worthy of adult attention. The chapter highlights the significant ways in which young children understand AIDS, sex, sexuality and the gendered narratives they deploy in relation to disease. Children's presumed innocence, the social (and sexual) construction of AIDS and the heterosexualisation of desire and danger are key themes which punctuate boys' and girls' narratives of AIDS. The sexual transmission of the disease provided children with ample opportunity to discuss boyfriends and girlfriends, kissing and playing heterosexual games as they contested and challenged each other as boys and girls. When children are given the opportunity and space to talk about AIDS, their investments in heterosexuality, desires and pleasures and their gendered narratives are made visible. Their sexual desires and pleasures, anxieties and fears were, to a greater or lesser extent, self-willed, whether adults approved or not. What this suggests is that given the right circumstances, children are very thoughtful and actively negotiate their own sexual predicaments, their pleasures and their concerns. Even at ages seven and eight, boys and girls are capable of reflecting on their actual lives and are happy to talk about AIDS and sexuality, but they are also acutely aware of being governed and controlled by discourses of innocence. How children resist and negotiate knowledge of the disease is discussed in Chapter 5. As Walkerdine (2004) suggests, recourse to notions of childhood innocence in pedagogic discourses has the effect of turning displays of sexuality into something that is hidden, forbidden and subverted. To act and talk sexually is a breach of order and a form of trouble in itself and young children know this and are remarkable agents in managing adult concerns and anxieties. The understanding of heterosexual behaviour and the pleasure; the use of the condom, as articulated by Donovan and the discussion of rape; and working-class girls' vulnerability to HIV, suggested by Thobeka and Gugu, are dangerous knowledge, particularly in the context of childhood innocence. Working-class femininities are constructed within the spectre of fear (both real and imagined), and the girls inscribe themselves within this discourse and reinvent the rampant African male sexuality in South Africa (Pendry 1998). Their understandings of male violence must be situated within a broader context where the experience of and fear related to rape is real.

Children are already inserting within dominant understandings of gender, sexuality and disease in ways that could create further vulnerability in the future. Children's AIDS-related knowledge is very messy and invokes fear and danger, laughter and pleasure and distance and othering. In order to take children seriously, children need to have access to broader knowledge systems to build their understandings of disease whilst paying attention to their active participation in sexual cultures and gendered asymmetries of power. As Robinson (2013) suggests in reimagining childhood, adults need to accept children as sexual subjects that take children's sexuality seriously as they do other aspects of their being whilst promoting, recognising and valuing their agency, and their right as gendered and sexual agents. In order to begin counteracting the threat to young children, there is need broadening the scope of young children's knowledge of AIDS that demands a rethink of childhood innocence, their vulnerability and their sexual and health well-being more widely.

## REFERENCES

Allen, L. (2014) 'Don't Forget, Thursday Is Test[icle] Time! The Use of Humour in Sexuality Education'. *Sex Education*, 14(4): 387–399.

Bhana, D. & Epstein, D. (2007) ' "I Don't Want to Catch It" Boys, Girls and Sexualities in an HIV Environment'. *Gender and Education*, 19(1): 109–125.

Blaise, M. (2010) 'Kiss and Tell: Gendered Narratives in Childhood Sexuality'. *Australasian Journal of Early Childhood*, 35(1): 1–9.

Epstein, D. & Johnson, R. (1998) *Schooling Sexualities*. Buckingham: Open University Press.

Epstein, D., O'Flynn, S. & Telford, D. (2003) *Silenced Sexualities in Schools and Universities*. Stoke-on-Trent: Trentham Books.

Hey, V. (1997) *The Company She Keeps: An Ethnography of Girls' Friendships*. Buckingham: Open University Press.

Hunter, M. (2005) 'Cultural Politics and Masculinities: Multiple-Partners in Historical Perspective in KwaZulu-Natal'. *Culture, Health and Sexuality*, 7: 389–403.

Pendry, B. (1998) 'The Links Between Gender Violence and HIV/AIDS'. *Agenda*, 39: 30–33.

Robinson, K. (2013) *Innocence, Knowledge and the Construction of Childhood: The Contradictory Nature of Sexuality and Censorship in Children's Contemporary Lives Contemporary Lives*. New York: Routledge.

Robinson, K. H. (2005) 'Childhood and Sexuality: Adult Constructions and Silenced Children', in J. Mason & T. Fattore (eds) *Children Taken Seriously in Theory, Policy and Practice* (pp. 66–78). London: Jessica Kingsley.

Shisana, O., Rehle, T., Simbayi, L.C., Zuma, K., Jooste, S., Zungu, N. (2014) *South African National HIV Prevalence, Incidence and Behaviour Survey, 2012*. Cape Town: HSRC Press.

Thamm, M. (2002) *I Have Life: Alison's Journey as Told to Marianne Thamm*. Johannesburg: The Penguin Group.

Thorne, B. (1993) *Gender Play: Girls and Boys in School*. Brunswick: Rutgers University Press.

Walkerdine, V. (2004) 'Development Psychology and the Study of Childhood', in M. Kehily (ed) *An Introduction to Childhood Studies* (pp. 96–107). Buckingham: Open University Press.

# 3 AIDS and Stigma
## Race, Class, Gender, Sexuality and Inequalities in Children's Response to Disease

> If you don't want to catch AIDS, you stay away from people that
> have AIDS. Even if they don't have cuts, you just stay away . . .
> Like if you did not want to catch it, I would not go near somebody
> that had it!
>
> —Conversation with eight-year old Catherine in grade two
> at Bullwood Primary School

The children in this chapter emerge from Bullwood, where HIV prevalence rates are low but where AIDS ties people together whether rich or poor. The sexual transmission of AIDS, and its rooting in the social cultural context in the country, is an eloquent testimony to the salience of the links between rich and poor. Young white children might not see AIDS in their families, but they know of AIDS, they hear about it through their social environments (e.g. through death and illness of domestic workers in their homes), and they hear about it in church, on radio, on television and through massive visual and other representations of AIDS prevention messages posted throughout the country. The AIDS pandemic, despite the racialised construction of the disease as black and other (Petros *et al.* 2006), is a striking reminder of the links between poverty and plenty.

As researchers we need to be able to see children's AIDS-related knowledge from multiple directions, from different vantage points and social contexts. As I have argued in Chapter 1, children's AIDS-related knowledge is produced within the everyday social life where sexuality, gender, race, class and age coalesce in the social production of the disease. Like Jackson and Scott (2010: 2), who locate the production of sexuality to the "mundane actualities of social life", children's knowledge of the disease cannot be separated from social life at Bullwood. In this chapter I am interested in the ways in which children's knowledge of AIDS is expressed in ways that are an outcome of these complex social processes. How children at Bullwood give meaning to AIDS is culturally and historically specific and embroiled in power. Children's meanings of AIDS are stitched into the very fabric of power and weave intricately with wider social relations both challenging and reproducing inequalities.

In this chapter, I show how children express knowledge of the disease through a complex well of inequalities reflective of the South African landscape—and highly stigmatising (Pulerwitz & Bongaarts 2014). Parker and Aggelton (2003) suggest that AIDS-related stigma is complexly connected to existing inequalities of race, gender and class and involves the language of power, inequality and exclusion. Showing how wider social representations and practices feed into stigmatisation of people with HIV/AIDS, South African scholars have contributed to the growing literature on stigma and the social exclusion of people with AIDS (Campbell *et al.* 2005, 2007; Kalichman *et al.* 2005; Shisana *et al.* 2005). A serious omission in this work is that it fails to seriously consider the divergent nature of responses to AIDS (Jewkes 2006). Discussions of HIV-related stigma usually draw on the now-classic work of Goffman (1963), who defines stigma as a "discrediting attribute" leading scholars to a focus on stigma as a static concept characterising people in unmediated ways, a criticism noted by Parker and Aggelton (2003). Notably absent from scholarly work in HIV-related stigma is a more nuanced understanding beyond simply the question of "what we do and how it is wrong" (ibid.: 2; see Norman *et al.* [2007] as an exception).

Applied to children, a nuanced conception of stigma rejects the search for some static logic in their responses to AIDS. Instead, it posits an understanding of children's account of AIDS as being constructed through self-regulation and contestation under specific social circumstances where material and cultural factors interact with popular understandings of contagion in mediating knowledge about the disease. This chapter shows how children struggle, adjust and confirm relations of power whilst going beyond stigma, inhabiting contradictorily a position of care and concern for those infected with AIDS. Showing how children use stigma in response to AIDS, it is influenced by the growing body of work on AIDS-related stigma which argues that stigma is not a static concept but ever changing and linked centrally to the social and economic power differentials that sculpt the meanings of the disease (Castro & Farmer 2005). These scholars note that stigma is invariably rooted in structural violence that generates social inequalities.

Large-scale social forces which define structural violence include poverty, racism, gender inequalities and physical violence, and these in turn are inextricably linked to the legacy of apartheid and the persistent economic processes and inequalities that shape the South African landscape (Hunter 2007). Rising unemployment, extensive geographical movement of men and women as a result of urbanisation and industrialisation coupled with the history of a migrant labour system have contributed to fragile family structures for the majority in the country. It matters who you are as a child and where you are in the experience of and vulnerability to AIDS. As I argued in Chapter 1 income distribution in South Africa remains highly unequal and racialised despite the end of apartheid, and the intimate ties with race and class persists, albeit with some changes to the emergence of an African elite. These complex social processes mark the distribution and outcomes of

AIDS in the country and have been particularly important in explaining why Africans and African women, in particular, have greater vulnerability to risk of infection, rate of disease progression and, in large part, remain the people who suffer from AIDS-related stigma and discrimination. Important scholarship has thus demonstrated that it is precisely the poor who are at greater risk for infection and more vulnerable than their wealthy counterparts (who remain largely white). Children too, as this chapter shows, not only insert meanings along the fault lines of economic and social structures that shape the South African landscape but also respond as subjects who show care and concern and who are also easily stigmatised for possessing sexual knowledge. Discourses of childhood innocence stigmatise and exclude those who do not conform to the ideals of innocence (Holland 2004). Innocence serves to reproduce the idea that children are separate from the sociocultural context in which they live, are blank sheets and are thus separate from gender, race, class or power (Tobin 1997). Breaking from these perspectives the new sociology of childhood drawing from post-structuralist perspectives argues that children are agents, positioned within particular discourses. Children despite dominating views about their innocence actively make meanings, protest, conform and navigate the social worlds in which they are located (Thorne 1993).

A number of researchers have begun to explore the context of AIDS related stigma in South Africa and comment on the social exclusion of people with AIDS (Campbell *et al.* 2005; Delius & Glaser 2005; Petros *et al.* 2006; Campbell *et al.* 2007). These studies, whilst exploring the multidimensional sources of AIDS, have been characterised by a central omission: a failure to take seriously the views and divergent responses of very young children in the construction of HIV-related stigma, an omission that goes beyond the continent. There is very little knowledge of how stigma is constructed and resisted by young children under specific social circumstances. Protecting children from risk and danger remains an overriding theme that informs many responses to children in vulnerable and development contexts (Chase & Aggleton 2006).

Exploring the manifestation of stigma in children's responses to AIDS, this chapter shows how boys and girls at Bullwood negotiate, construct and reproduce meaning about the disease and the discourses they deploy in so doing. Popular beliefs regarding AIDS as highly infectious or as "catchy", as the earlier quote illustrates, has played an important role in stigma and has remained steadfastly impervious to public health messages (Delius & Glaser 2005). Amidst the complexity of meanings that children harness in making meaning of the disease and the socially diverse responses to it, a central theme was that of 'catching it'. The idea of catchy germs is an important element of children's construction of stigma and was complexly articulated in children's responses around race, class, sex and gender. Whilst the sexual connection with the disease remains an important source of stigma, evidence suggests that popular understandings of contagion constitute a relatively unyielding and significant element in the multidimensional sources of AIDS-related stigma (Campbell *et al.* 2007). Young children's constitution of stigma—rarely featuring in AIDS research and debate—is not a straightforward process but, as this chapter shows, is deeply intertwined and tied to contagion and the reproduction of power inequalities.

## AIDS, STIGMA AND RACE

### Black Heterosexual Masculinity and Disease

A significant characteristic of HIV-related stigma is that the disease has to do with African people who are constructed as inherently diseased and promiscuous (McClintock 1995). Children's knowledge of African men as vectors in the spread of the disease was premised on their association and knowledge of African men and women who worked in their homes as domestic labourers:

> Dianne:   Bridget said that her maid died of AIDS, . . . that her boyfriend slept with one girl and made her pregnant and then came and slept with her.

In South Africa many scholars note how dominant African masculinities shape men's control over women and celebrate multiple partners that drive the gendered nature of the epidemic (Hunter 2005). In the preceding transcript, Dianne relates the circumstances surrounding Bridget's maid's death and points to multiple partnering as important in fuelling the HIV pandemic. What is significant here is that the girls are learning to recognise the vulnerabilities faced by women. As illustrated elsewhere, the girls in this study construct men as bad, pitting violent men against innocent women, but this was also highly racialised with African men being constructed as vectors in the spread of the disease, violent and feared (Bhana 2007). African men have been particularly problematised in the context of the HIV epidemic, with campaigns and literature addressing them, especially, as people with multiple partners who engage in forms of sexual harassment and violence.

The conversation about domestic work, however, not only provided access to knowledge about sex, death, disease and gender inequalities but also opened the conversation in ways that invoked fear of blood and contagion functioning to reproduce the racialised discourses under apartheid:

> Beatrice:   My aunt's house . . . at my aunt's house, there was this gardener and then he died of AIDS and his blood . . . when he was dying his blood was on the spade and then I went to play with it and my aunt said, "No don't touch it otherwise you might get AIDS like him!"

"Don't touch it" is emotionally powerful because it reproduces popular constructions and anxieties around contagion, as well as race and class. Unlike apartheid, however, the new equation of racism is also one that constructs Africans as AIDS vectors. Children's construction of race and AIDS-related stigma takes place in a web of competing access to meanings and symbols of representation of AIDS. Dianne's version of the disease suggests an understanding of AIDS as part of a network of relations that are economic (racial) and sexual breaking the myth of sexual innocence. Beatrice, however, locks into popular constructions of the disease as contagious, reproducing power inequalities.

## Race, Class and Disease

The next transcript shows that as HIV-related stigma is produced in relation to race, it does not happen in a transparent manner but involves disputations. Stigma is thus not some fixed entity but moving and shifting within the specific setting at Bullwood:

DB: Who gets AIDS?
Carver: Whites, blacks and Indians, everyone.
Allan: Mainly Africans.
DB: How do you know?
Allan: 'Cause I normally see it on TV that mainly Africans have it.
Blythe: Mostly I think that it's old people, around their forties and around their sixties.
Anne: No not really. I think more the black people. Babies get AIDS as well and mostly all the Africans that live on the street and stuff. They all get AIDS and that's how they catch it.

Poverty in South Africa is unequally distributed a point captured by Anne who constructs Africans as living "on the street and stuff" and catching AIDS, an experience that is quite different from middle-class white contexts. Taking issue with simple reproductionist accounts of AIDS-related stigma, the children's responses show how meanings about the vectors in the spread of the disease are being recreated. Carver suggests that "everyone" gets it. This is important particularly because it breaks down and rejects a homogenous construction of white people as racists and invulnerable to disease. "Whites, blacks and Indians" are all complicit in the spread of the disease and vulnerable. Another area of disputation involves age. Blythe is able to make the relationship between old age and death by inserting the dreaded disease as part of the explanation for death. In fact, an important theme that that developed in the study was the way in which children often associated the disease with death and old age some even suggesting that their grandparents had died of AIDS. Anne's construction of vulnerable babies draws directly from the steep rise in infection among women tested at antenatal clinics. In 2003, for example, 26.5% of women tested in antenatal clinics were HIV positive (Department of Health 2005), and this has had a grave impact on the number of babies born with the disease. Taken together, children do not simply insert into apartheid-defined racism. AIDS-related stigma and race are constructed within a context of adjustment and contestation showing a great deal of sophistication but also inserting within racist discourses. Allan's point highlights the statistical fact in South Africa "mainly Africans have it", a fact that he draws from the media representation of AIDS in South Africa. The ways in which the media represents AIDS is important particularly in the South African context in which African people receive a great deal of attention suggesting how some people are and are not at risk. Clearly, African people—as Allan points out—have received media coverage in the spread of AIDS, whilst Shisana and Simbayi (2002) suggest that black South Africans are more likely to be infected with the disease than whites (12.9% compared to 6.2%). Socio-economic status is an important co-factor in the spread of the disease. Economic hardship and social exclusion work to create vulnerability to HIV infection and to the stigmatisation of the African poor, who are more vulnerable to infection in South Africa.

> Nicole:    Some blacks dig in the black bags and eat all the rotten food and they think it's okay to eat it and they won't get sick but they do.
>
> Jan:    *Ja*, I saw this one man when I was riding, um, in my car with my mom and dad and my brother. We went past this black bag and there was a black man next to it and he was eating a banana peel . . . a banana peel yes.
>
> DB:    Are black people spreading AIDS?
>
> Nicole:    I don't know, just germs. They have germs, they don't have cream, they don't have everything else to keep their bodies clean, all that.
>
> Delia:    I don't know.

Collectively the children associated HIV infection with dirt and disease and located it in the lower socio-economic groups—and these are mainly African contexts. When I asked about the disease, a common response was "Some blacks are getting it". Children were generally critical of black people, distancing themselves from what they perceived to be permissive sexuality and erecting racial barriers and reinforcing racial types typical of apartheid South Africa.

These children had clearly learned to associate AIDS with black people, dirt, germs and poverty. While it is true that AIDS disproportionately affects black people and is socially constructed through race and class, the children struggled to give meaning to these social constructs. There is a great deal of ambiguity in the above conversation, which brings together potent symbols of dirt, disease, racism, infection and stigma.

The fear of germs and the contempt for the unsanitary behaviour of the poor (and African people) that the children expressed do not simply reproduce racialised identities and distancing but also suggest the discursive mechanisms that young children deploy in managing their own concerns and anxieties. Nicole and Delia banish AIDS to the domain of poor Africans and thus distance themselves from poverty, disease and the other. Unlike the racist tropes on African sexuality that exaggerate the importance of sex in the spread of AIDS, the children drew on disease, poverty and hunger—all co-factors of HIV infection—to reproduce a racist stereotype. Young children's understanding of the disease is thus created through systems of representation that work on the broader social and cultural differences in South Africa.

These differences work to constrain and create meaning in ambiguous ways. However, the girls were not confident that black people were responsible for spreading AIDS, Nicole's reference to germs and Delia's statement "I don't know" suggest this.

The next lengthy conversation with Diane and Beate suggests how magic, sorcery and witchcraft come together in stigmatising Africans:

> Diane:   . . . [S]ome people, they actually want to give other people AIDS and like kill them. And they actually take them to the witchdoctor and they kill the people at the witchdoctor and they take their blood and make a special potion and that potion is in us and they make other people get AIDS and very sick 'cause they are taking the blood to make juice or something and people drink that from the shops and they actually get very bad AIDS, so it likes kills them and the people that have AIDS they catch them again and they take the blood from them and make everyone get more and more AIDS and give it to every single person and people get more and more AIDS . . .

How do we understand Diane's representation of AIDS and the association with witchcraft, sorcery and race? In the context where children like Diane neither experience AIDS nor get information about the disease the idea that AIDS is spread by the magical powers of witchdoctors is perhaps unsurprising. Taking a cue from Treichler (1999) it is argued here that even children are able to make sense of the disease, even imperfectly, reproducing conspiracy and racialised views that have social and historical specificity, as they try to understand the terrifying phenomenon of AIDS. Not all children subscribed to this view, and even within the same school context there were discrepant views, but in this section, I am interested in demonstrating the variation of meanings as it "serves as templates for the charged social divisions and power inequalities" (Treichler 1999: 220). Diane continues and goes on to associate AIDS with the evil *ubuthakathi*, linking it to blood and violence, and this is highly racialised:

DB: What are witchdoctors?

Diane: Well they have like sharp knives and they are Africans and some are whites, but there are not so many white ones like one or two or something, but mostly they are African ones. They take people's blood and like spray things on them and take their blood and they drink it and those people like get stronger and stronger. They steal things and sell them and then pay the shops to put their juices in the shops and like they steal knives to kill people with it and they like steal jewellery 'cause the witchdoctor she or whatever has got rings all over her hands and like lots of necklaces . . .

Beate: No they don't have much powers, like no powers, but they have potion made out of blood and all kinds of stuff that they put on people like maybe like their heart or something like that and they get ugly like grey things that they eat . . . They mix all the things together . . . They actually catch about, they get like five people who don't have AIDS and they die. Then they take all those people and take all their blood and they get like five pups and maybe more and full of blood. And they take, maybe their hearts . . . and blood from those people and . . . they take little bit from that person and that person and that person and they put it all in the same pot and they mix it all up and then they take like different blood and mix it in there . . .

Historical evidence shows how selected body parts removed from deceased people were used to enhance magical powers amongst isiZulu (McClendon 2006), much to the condemnation of colonial forces who subjected those who killed in the name of witchcraft to punitive laws, including the removal of cattle (most prized economic possession). Beate and Diane are excited as they incite the horror of AIDS, linking it with blood, magical potions, body parts (the heart), race and crime. The representation of AIDS is evil with African people and, is connected with the spread of the disease in magical ways: infecting, mixing blood, putting their juices in shops and inciting further the terror in the spread of AIDS. AIDS conspiracy theories circulate geographically (Natrass 2013), and what is being recirculated here is a local conspiracy that Africans, in particular with their use of potions and magical powers associated with blood, violence and crime and the spread AIDS with terrifying descriptions of bloodthirsty monsters.

This is a racialised pattern. Africans do bear the brunt of the disease, and in giving credence to the theory of the witchdoctor, Diane and Beate extend the racial divide, separate from the disease and distance themselves from Africans and AIDS. The association with AIDS and witchdoctors reproduces long-standing historical and racialised structures of meaning in which nascent representation of the disease is embedded. Even at ages seven and eight, young children are able to make sense of AIDS deploying conspiracy theories that have historical and local relevance. Natrass (2013: 2) argues that AIDS conspiracy theories are "invented and shaped by agents". As agents in the social construction of AIDS, young children invent and put together a variety of ideas—blood, magic, witchdoctors, race, history, class, violence, crime—to forge a racialised and specific theory about AIDS based on conspiracy.

## Race, Disease and Care

This part of the section shows how care emerges and permeates children's racialised construction of the disease. Jewkes (2006) asserts that progression of HIV infection to AIDS has made the disease a painful and visible reality for many in South Africa. The children in this study know about AIDS through a variety of sources having knowledge of it through information about their domestic workers, from the media or being warned to stay away from blood. But they also know about AIDS through their churches:

> Ashleigh:  When we went down to valley with our church, 'cause every time we go there, usually every second weekend, to see poor children that live in the valley and have AIDS and sickness like that, we give them presents like sweets, and we have this little girl, she was born like a few weeks ago. She's three months old and she had AIDS and we then tried. We tried and we gave all these milk bottles and dummies and stuff like that and then, then a few weeks later she died.
>
> DB:  What's down the valley?
>
> Alex:  It's called a place down the road and there are lots of people that have AIDS there.
>
> DB:  How do you know that?
>
> Alex:  We go to church and we go help the people with AIDS and give them bread and stuff.

In the fight against AIDS, the South African government has appealed to all its constituencies to help combat the spread of the disease. The church is a significant religious institution working to help preach messages that help prevent behaviour that increases risk to infection but is also actively involved in care. Ashleigh and Alex point out this fact that they, too, are involved in assisting those infected. The transcripts illustrate the ways that AIDS provides the intimate link between rich and poor through the production of discourses of care challenging the instrumental accounts of AIDS-related stigma. Children are not only inserting within specific social processes and actively producing inequalities but they also insert within discourses of care. Ashleigh spoke with a great deal of sensitivity and concern about the baby that had died of AIDS—despite "dummies, milk bottles, sweets and presents" the baby died. AIDS has produced a climate of not only distancing but also of connecting social environments where communities and children are becoming familiar with illness, death and pain. The next transcript reinforces this argument and shows how children show concern and care for orphans:

> Alistair: They [African children] don't have TV too. They don't have TV to know about AIDS and they don't have their mothers and fathers and their mothers and fathers haven't had TVs in their lives so they probably don't know about AIDS.
>
> Natalie: And maybe they don't even have their moms and dads so their moms and dads can't tell them.
>
> DB: Where are their moms and dads?
>
> Natalie: I think that, I don't know, maybe their moms and dads died.
>
> Alistair: Maybe they're orphans.
>
> Charles: Because they are always out on the streets and all the germs are out on the streets and they have sores . . .
>
> Alistair: . . . [T]hey have no homes, they live on the streets, and they got no money so they can't buy pills or medicines so they can't, so they get sick easily . . .

The children in this study show why the concept of stigma as a static unidirectional process has little meaning when applied to their lives. It is far more complex and is embedded within increasingly divergent social responses illustrating care and concern and showing how poverty and lack of access to information about AIDS (as on the TV) increases vulnerability to disease and germs. The children are painfully aware of death of parents and the many orphans in South Africa. UNICEF (2007) has urged South Africa to do much more to raise awareness of AIDS amid rising child deaths. AIDS is the leading cause of child mortality and accounts for between 40% and 60% of all deaths nationwide. As the conversation took on a serious frame, children suggested ways of helping people with AIDS, displacing the irrational concerns about contagion to sharing food and drinks with those infected but these emergent responses are also situated ambiguously within a context where power inequalities are being reproduced:

> Jenna: You can give them special pills and make them feel happy.
>
> Storm: You can say nice things about them.
>
> DB: What else can you do?
>
> Adam: You can share your food with them and your drinks.
>
> Jenna: They should go have a special treatment done or something.
>
> Storm: *Ja*, they should like go to a kind of place where they like help people with AIDS and make them happy and stuff.
>
> David: Maybe they can go to the side of the road and beg for food and money. Find a job or something and don't live in shacks!

> Storm: Some people find like paper or cardboard and they like write stuff like "Please help me I have AIDS and I need some money please. Give me a job".
>
> David: Once I read a sign, this one guy said, "Please give me a home".
>
> Jenna: Some people live in bushes, grass and stuff like that.

Discourses of care do not stand outside the systems of representation that work on the broader social and cultural differences in South Africa. On one hand, the conversation shows care and concern. Jenna, Adam and Storm suggest sharing drinks (despite the hegemony of contagion in children's conversations) and show concern about the happiness of HIV-infected people. David shifts the conversation drawing attention to the rising unemployment in South Africa, which sees many African men hold up signs pleading for jobs and begging for food. He displaces the conversation from care to the reproduction of power inequalities and shows contempt for the lives and experiences of the poor who beg and who live in "shacks"—often described as informal African township settlements clustered around urban areas. Informal settlements have HIV rates of infection almost twice as high as urban and rural areas (Pettifor *et al.* 2004). By locking into intersecting relations of power, the children move the conversation from care to contempt of people considered different—poor, black shack dwellers, the unemployed and the diseased.

## AIDS, STIGMA AND SEXUALITY

### AIDS—the Gay Disease

The following transcript shows the competing narratives through which AIDS as the gay disease becomes visible. The role of contagion features in the accounts of AIDS as a gay disease:

> Michael: You don't have to play with someone to get AIDS. You can get AIDS anywhere. Like in the news like, there's 50 or 100 ways of getting AIDS. I know that there is some way to get AIDS. The thing that I know about how to get AIDS is that you touch someone's blood and spit on someone, if you are lesbian or what you call two boys? Like two boys or girls? [laughs]
>
> Andrew: Gay [laughs], Gross!
>
> Sarah: *Ja*, gay. I won't kiss a girl!
>
> Michael: If they're [gays] having sex with someone or like sex or some drugs. I know that those are the things like 20 or so things. As you get bigger, you learn more and more about AIDS.

The popular script of contagion in the spread of the disease is displaced because Michael disputes contagion as route of transmission. Yet he reinserts within such popular scripts of contagion as he refers to spitting as a route of transmission before he suggests explicit knowledge of sex and drugs. However, gay sex becomes a visible marker of disease. The children in this study know about sex and AIDS in variable ways (see Bhana 2007), but their sexuality is also caught up and normalised in the processes of heterosexuality. In the earlier vignette, dominant notions of heterosexuality involve the projection of an abiding heterosexual self, which is related to homophobia. As the boys and girls give meaning to AIDS, they also do so in ways that are gendered and sexual. Andrew's and Sarah's words "gross" and "I won't kiss a girl" are illustrative of the making of heterosexual gendered identities. Andrew establishes a heterosexual grounding by publicly asserting the non-normative ways of sexuality, defiling gayness through contempt. Sarah's "I won't kiss a girl" not only suggests knowledge of sexual activity but also confirms the power invested in the heterosexual norm and the repulsion associated with gay kissing. Even for children of this age, the pressure for heteronormativity is present and has an impact on how the disease is viewed in a country where heterosexuality is the chief form of infection. The visibility of AIDS as a gay disease is thus interconnected with the production of normalised masculinities and femininities through the heterosexual regulation. In giving meaning to AIDS as a gay disease, complex processes intersect where boys and girls attempt to get their gender right. Rejecting the idea of AIDS as exclusively a gay disease Michael suggests that there are 20, 50 or 100 ways of getting AIDS, which, he adds, can be learnt as children get "bigger". Age dynamics are evident marking out the boundaries of how much and when children have the right to such knowledge. Whilst Michael broke down the myth of childhood innocence by making explicit reference to sex, he was also positioning himself as a child (and thus less knowledgeable) and without the same right to knowledge about the disease. In Chapter 5 I also explore further what this means in terms of heterosexual kissing, boyfriends and girlfriends.

## CONCLUSION

In this chapter, I have drawn attention to the issue of AIDS-related stigma in relation to the young children. It has shown that AIDS-related stigma has deep social roots connected to race, class, gender, age and sexuality. The chapter has also drawn attention to the issue of contagion that manifest in the AIDS response. Going beyond the simple reproduction of power inequalities, the chapter shows the sophisticated ways in which children navigate the context of HIV, not only involving intense self-regulatory practices, confirming and resisting power inequalities but also disposed to patterns of care and concern. This has profound implications for efforts to stem the spread of AIDS-related stigma and discrimination in South Africa, because it highlights the contradictory discursive contexts within which young children give meaning to stigma.

Children's articulation of stigma occurs at the nexus of great structural inequalities and requires a massive transformation of the South African landscape that predisposes the majority to HIV risk and stigma. The South African government is hard at work in its attempt to address structural inequalities. Yet as the United Nations Development Programme (2003) report suggests, much more has to be done with this regard particularly in a context where striking inequalities are pervasive. There is a great deal of political will to redress these inequalities particularly as the post-apartheid context has enshrined rights, democracy and equality. The work has just begun, and there is much more to do.

For both political/democratic and health reasons, it would appear evident that finding ways to address issues of AIDS-related stigma at an age at which the children's right to AIDS education has often been neglected could offer a way forward. AIDS education is compulsory for all South African children beginning from the first stages of formal schooling, and yet for all its efforts to ensure equality and abolish discrimination, the early stages of children's lives have received very little attention (Department of Education 1999). Much has been written about the inefficacy of education in addressing stigma (Brown *et al.* 2003) as well as the inability of education to do this alone (Campbell *et al.* 2007). Whilst the question about education's role in addressing stigma remains complex, in early childhood education the work has yet to begin. Discourses of children's innocence and dominant ideas of children's incompetence around serious matters like AIDS are pervasive (Bhana 2007). Children have very few opportunities with adults (both parents and teachers) to talk openly about the disease despite the educational policy. To assume that children do not know about the disease (or are too young to know) and therefore cannot, or do not, engage with the disease is simplistic, decontextualised from larger social processes and a shallow representation of the sophisticated way that children engage with their social worlds (James *et al.* 1998). Putting the young person first, promoting the participation of the child and addressing issues around social justice and equality within the specific context of the young person's social circumstance (see Chase & Aggleton 2006) are key to understanding the complex mediation of AIDS-related stigma and developing strategies to combat stigma. Efforts to address young children as active agents in making sense of stigma in the context of AIDS must begin and increase, requiring greater vigilance and care for the lives of young children from parents and educational stakeholders. Stigma is more likely to thrive in environments of ignorance and half-truths (Valdiserri 2002). Children must have knowledge of the disease about how it is spread and how it is not transmitted, ensuring that taboo subjects of sexuality feature in such discussions. This will also require that adults (whether teachers or parents) provide an environment where they can talk to children in ways that recognise them as subjects in struggle who are sexual, gendered, as well as race and class defined. Greater efforts are needed not only to address the negative effects of AIDS-related stigma but also to work and build on the positive insights that young children bring in making sense of stigma.

# REFERENCES

Bhana, D. (2007) 'Childhood Sexualities and Rights in HIV Contexts'. *Culture Health and Sexuality*, 9(3): 309–324.

Brown, L., Macintyre, K. & Trujillo, T. (2003) 'Interventions to Reduce HIV-Related Stigma: What Have We Learned'. *AIDS Education & Prevention*, 15: 49–69.

Campbell, C., Foullis, C. A., Maimane, S. & Sibiya, Z. (2005) ' "I Have an Evil Child at My House". Stigma and HIV/AIDS Management in a South African Community'. *American Journal of Public Health*, 95: 808–815.

Campbell, C., Nair, Y., Maimane, S. & Nicholson, J. (2007) 'A Multi-Level Model of Roots in HIV-Related Stigma in Two South African Communities'. *Journal of Health Psychology*, 12(3): 403–416.

Castro, A. & Farmer, P. (2005) 'Understanding and Addressing HIV-Related Stigma: From Anthropological Theory to Clinical Practice in Haiti'. *American Journal of Public Health*, 95(1): 53–59.

Chase, E. & Aggleton, P. (2006) 'Meeting the Sexual Health Needs of Young People Living on the Street', in R. Ingham & P. Aggleton (eds) *Promoting Young People's Sexual Health* (pp. 81–98). London: Routledge.

Delius, P. & Glaser, C. (2005) 'Sex, Disease and Stigma in South Africa: Historical Perspectives'. *African Journal of AIDS Research*, 4(1): 29–36.

Department of Education. (1999) *Revised National Curriculum Statement Grade R-9 Life Orientation*. Pretoria: Department of Education.

Department of Health. (2005) *Summary Report: National HIV and Syphilis Antenatal Sero-Prevalence Survey in South Africa 2002*. Department of Health, Health Systems Research, Research Coordination and Epidemiology, Republic of South Africa.

Goffman, E. (1963) *Stigma: Notes on the Management of Spoiled Identity*. Englewood Cliffs, NJ: Prentice Hall.

Holland, P. (2004) *Picturing Childhood: The Myth of the Child in Popular Imagery*. London: I. B. Tauris.

Hunter, M. (2005) 'Cultural Politics and Masculinities: Multiple-Partners in Historical Perspective in KwaZulu-Natal'. *Culture, Health and Sexuality*, 7: 389–403.

Hunter, M. (2007) 'The Changing Political Economy of Sex in South Africa: The Significance of Unemployment and Inequalities to the Scale of the AIDS Pandemic'. *Social Science & Medicine*, 64(3): 689–700.

Jackson, S. & Scott, S. (2010) *Theorizing Sexuality*. Maidenhead: McGraw-Hill/Open University Press.

James, A., Jencks, C. & Prout, A. (1998) *Theorising Childhood*. Cambridge: Polity.

Jewkes, R. (2006) 'Beyond Stigma: Social Responses to HIV in South Africa'. *The Lancet*, 368(9534): 430–431.

Kalichman, S. C., Simbayi, L. C., Jooste, S., Toefy, Y., Dain, D., Cherry, C. & Kagee, A. (2005) 'Development of a Brief Scale to Measure AIDS-Related Stigma in South Africa'. *AIDS Behaviour*, 9: 35–143.

McClendon, T. (2006) 'You Are What You Eat Up: Deposing Chiefs in Early Colonial Natal, 1847–58'. *The Journal of African History*, 47: 259–279.

McClintock, A. (1995) *Imperial Leather: Race, Gender and Sexuality in the Colonial Conquest*. London: Routledge.

Natrass, N. (2013) 'Understanding the Origins and Prevalence of AIDS Conspiracy Beliefs in the United States and South Africa', *Sociology of Health and Illness*,35(1):113-29.Norman, A., Chopra, M. A. & Kadiyala, S. (2007) 'Factors Related to HIV Disclosure in 2 South African Communities'. *American Journal of Public Health*, 97(10): 1775–1781.

Parker, R. & Aggleton, P. (2003) 'AIDS-Related Stigma and Discrimination: A Conceptual Framework and Implications for Action'. *Social Science & Medicine*, 57: 13–24.

Petros, G., Airhihenbuwa, H., Simbayi, L., Ramlagan, S. & Brown, B. (2006) 'HIV/AIDS and 'Othering' in South Africa: The Blame Goes On'. *Culture Health and Sexuality*, 8(1): 67–77.

Pettifor, A. E., Rees, H. V., Steffenson, A., Hlongwa-Madikizela, L., Macphail, C., Vermaak, K. & Kleinschmidt, I. (2004) *HIV and Sexual Behaviour Among Young South Africans: National Survey of 15–24 Year-Olds*. Reproductive Health Research Unit, University of Witwatersrand, Johannesburg.

Pulerwitz, J., & Bongaarts, J (2014). 'Tackling Stigma: Fundamental to an AIDS-Free Future'. *The Lancet Global Health*, 2(6): e311–e312.

Shisana, O., Rehle, T. & Simbayi, L. C. (2005) *South African National HIV Prevalence, HIV Incidence, Behaviour and Communication Survey*. Cape Town: Human Sciences Research Council.

Shisana, O. & Simbayi, L. (2002) *South African National HIV Prevalence, Behavioural Risks and Mass Media Household Survey*. Cape Town: HSRC Publishers.

Thorne, B. (1993) *Gender Play: Girls and Boys in School*. New Brunswick: Rutgers University Press.

Tobin, J. (ed). (1997) *Making a Place for Pleasure in Early Childhood Education*. New Haven, CT: Yale University Press.

Treichler, P. A. (1999) *How to Have Theory in an Epidemic: Cultural Chronicles of AIDS*. Durham, NC: Duke University Press.

UNICEF. (2007) *Progress for Children: A World Fit for Children Statistical Review* (No. 6). New York: UNICEF.

United Nations Development Programme. (2003) *South African Human Development Report 2003*. Oxford: Oxford University Press.

Valdiserri, R. O. (2002) 'HIV-Related Stigma: An Impediment to Public Health'. *American Journal of Public Health*, 92: 341–342.

# 4  "AIDS Is Rape!" Gender and Sexuality in Children's Responses to AIDS

Fezile:      From rape you get AIDS.
Gugu:        AIDS is rape . . .
DB:          What's rape?
Nokulunga:   When and older person calls you and does bad things to you.
Mlondi:      A person grabs you when you are going to the shops and then does bad things to you.
Nontobeko:   When he's doing bad things to you . . . he puts his penis in you with force . . .

—Focus group discussion with young African children aged between seven and eight in a working-class township context of *KwaDabeka*, Greater Durban, South Africa

How is AIDS interpreted and made meaningful by seven- and eight-year-old children at KwaDabeka? This present chapter focuses exclusively on the township school called KwaDabeka Primary School, and this backdrop provides contextual specificity to the meanings that African children give to the disease. Exploring the saliency of gender and sexuality in young African children's account of AIDS, this chapter shows how boys and girls construct meanings of the disease and the discourses they deploy in so doing. Risk of exposure to HIV, as young children begin to attest to, is related to a complex link involving sexual violence, highly unequal gender relations and age hierarchies. Children's understandings of AIDS are constructed through a range of social processes, and these forms of social relations frame their responses to the disease. Gender and sexual violence form a major focus in this chapter.

South Africa has the worst statistics on gender and sexual violence in the world. At least one in three South African women will be raped in her lifetime, and one in four will be beaten by her domestic partner (Jewkes *et al.* 2002). Moffett (2006) elucidates that the high rate of rape has fueled the pandemic in South Africa. About 20,000 girls between the ages of 0 and 17 are raped and reported to the police each year with adult males more often the perpetrators (Jewkes *et al.* 2005). Jewkes *et al.* (2002) found that 1.6% of a sample of more than 11,000 women had been raped before turning 15 years. Younger girls face greater biological susceptibility to HIV through vaginal mucosa, for example. It is widely known that what actually defines rape is variable and dependent on people's views of their experiences. South African law includes in its definition of rape penetration, non-consensual sex and the use of force and threats (Jewkes & Abrahams 2002). What actually constitutes rape, however, is far more complicated and depends for example on the age of those involved, social notions of gender roles as well as the relationship between the victim and the perpetrator. Wood, Lambert and Jewkes's (2007) study of African township men and women vividly illustrates this complexity. They argue that within local South African contexts, forced sex, unlike its legal definition, is a culturally expected form of male persuasion in romantic sexual relationships. Other scholars have noted that sexual violence in South African settings must be understood within a context of entrenched ideas about male privilege, as well as in terms of social inequalities, unemployment and deprivation amongst generations of black South African men, leading to greater vulnerability for women and girls (Jewkes *et al.* 2014). Woven together, sexual violence and HIV risk are deeply imbricated with gender and social inequalities. The sexual transmission of HIV, as young African children illustrated earlier, is testimony to the salience of these links.

In reconfiguring the passive and marginalized image of the young African child, in this chapter I draw attention to young children's active participation in unravelling the sexual and gender dynamics of AIDS. Young children are positioned as active agents with the capacity to engage with the disease and as agents who know and think around matters pertaining to gender and sexuality. Rejecting the view that children are incompetent and passive recipients of knowledge, the new sociology of childhood argues that children are competent interpreters of their world (Alderson 2007). In relation to gender and sexuality, evidence from the west shows how very young children in give meaning to sexuality through imaginative games, through laughter and exclamations, not only through conversations about kissing, boyfriends and girlfriends and going out but also through disgust, name-calling and the use of abusive language to those who do not fit normative and moral understandings of sexuality (Thorne 1993; Renold 2005; Robinson 2013). Such practices are means through which sexuality is expressed, shared and regulated.

The conceptualisation of the agency of African children, although marginal in both theory and debate, is not new in the African context. Historical perspectives in South Africa point to the dynamic and nuanced construction of sexuality and childhood. In precolonial South Africa, for example, Delius and Glaser (2002, 2005) argue that the association between children and sexuality was relatively open. Children often played sexual games without censure with sexual exploration being encouraged, monitored by peer groups and regulated. Sexualised games played by young children have been a longstanding feature of normal childhood (Jewkes *et al.* 2006). Scholars point to different historical moments and contexts in which sex play was a strong feature of African childhoods (that sometimes includes penetration as very common amongst girls and boys from about six or seven until early teenage years (Mager 1999). Importantly, the learning of sex was not frowned on even as it was monitored and regulated. Sex play remains an important currency in young African children's cultural worlds despite the adult wish to deny it (Bhana & Epstein 2007). Under the onslaught of Christianity, colonialism, urbanization, migration and ongoing cultural shifts the views about children and sexuality are mutating where dominating models sees the entrenching of masculinities which demand flesh-to-flesh sex, a celebration of multiple partners and the commodification and control over women and girls (Delius & Glaser 2002). Children are caught up in the crucible of HIV, sexual and gender violence and the meanings they attach to the disease reflect their vulnerability, their agency and their constraints.

Critiquing the muting of gender and sexuality this chapter foregrounds the ability of young children to exercise their agency. It focuses on AIDS, gender and sexuality and demonstrates how these factors inflect in the process of giving meaning to the disease. Young children's understandings of AIDS are the effects of material and discursive forces, although not determined by these social forces. They contest gender relations, confirm unequal gender inequalities and negotiate such meanings.

Understanding the ways in which gender and sexuality feature in children's responses to AIDS is crucial not only for the achievement of gender equality but is especially significant in developing prevention and educational programmes. Prevention programmes located firmly within sociocultural contexts in which young people are raised will better inform interventions that could instil, for example, habits and behaviours appropriate to their continued health and well-being in the context of the disease. Such programmes must start early and can only be determined by understanding the meanings that young people have constructed about AIDS. As Chong, Hallman and Brady (2006) argue, investing in young people is critical despite the fact that most researchers tend to shy away from sensitive topics including sexuality either because of social norms concerning age as well as doubts about the validity of young people's responses.

The rest of the chapter focuses on the ways that children give meaning to gender, sexuality and AIDS which is expressive of their contexts, their agency and their patterns of vulnerability.

## AIDS: SEX IS NAUGHTY

Children's elucidation of gender and sexuality in creating patterns of vulnerability to and experience of AIDS is a dominant theme. The accumulated effect of social violence, the burden of the disease embedded within highly unequal gender relations give rise to arguments that sexuality in Africa especially for women and girls is associated with pain and suffering not pleasure (Reddy 2004). Sex, as it shall be shown here, was not limited to this association. Drawing on the construction of sex as naughty the children (both boys and girls) inserted contradictorily within sexuality, framing it within the vocabulary of naughtiness imbuing it with negativity even as they derived pleasure in reporting on it. Children have an indefatigable curiosity about sex (Renold 2005). Through constant laughter and giggles, sexuality was framed as an area of embarrassment and laughter. Nayak and Kehily's (2001) work in schools in the United Kingdom show that laughter is an important area in understanding the projection of heterosexual desire among young people. The conversation that follows for example was loaded with giggles, smiles and laughter as children talked about heterosexual activity framing it as consensual, locating the toilet as a space for sexual activities whilst also linking it to the realm of naughtiness (and inappropriateness):

| | |
|---|---|
| DB: | How do you get AIDS? |
| Bongeka: | When people are naughty! [Giggles] |
| Zibuyile: | They take off their clothes and have sex. [laughter] |
| DB: | What is sex? |
| Zibuyile: | Kissing. |
| Thuso (b): | It's when you are going to make a child. |
| Nhlanhla (b): | That's being naughty. |
| Zibuyile: | It's a girl and boy sleeping together. [laughter] |
| DB: | What's being naughty? |
| Nhlanhla (b): | They climb on top of each other. |

Through their constructions of AIDS the children were giving meaning to sex and expressing it through laughter and giggles, presenting and asserting themselves as subjects with rights to knowledge about sex (Blaise 2010). As they speak up and out about AIDS they connect sex in pleasurable ways but paradoxically cast it as naughty and imbue it with negativity:

| | |
|---|---|
| DB: | What's sex? |
| Nokulunga: | It's being naughty. [laughter] |
| DB: | What's being naughty? |
| Nokulunga: | You go to the toilet and you do naughty things. |
| DB: | How? |
| Nokulunga: | A boy puts his penis inside a girl . . . When a boy calls a girl then they go to the toilet together. Then they go to the toilet to talk . . . Usually they whisper so that none can hear them. [laughter] |
| DB: | At schools—they go to the toilets? |
| Nokulunga: | Even at home it happens. There's one child who comes to KwaDabeka. |

| DB: | How do you know this? |
|---|---|
| Nokulunga: | I saw him. |
| DB: | Where? Were you at school? |
| Nokulunga: | No, at home in *bhuti* [elder person] Bonga's toilet. Then they closed the door so that nobody could see them. Then we opened it with my little sister. I said, "Yeye!" Then they ran away and Sane cried. We told her [Sane's] mother and she said she's going to smack her. |

The toilet is a sexualised space and a site for sexual expression and regulation. Against the backdrop of chronic overcrowding and deep poverty and in the context of one-room *imijondolos*, the narrative around sex as naughty is caught up in the space of the toilet and is the effect of material realities. The children in this study know sex and witness it. They emerge from one-room shacks where sexual activity takes place, but they also have knowledge that the toilet is often a more 'private' space where people can engage more intimately. Sane and her boyfriend, from the earlier testimony, position the toilet as a space where young people engage consensually. Nokulunga frames this sexual encounter within the space of the hidden, arousing sexuality as a silencing (sexual "whisperings") as well as the toilet as a space for sexual expression. The toilet in the township functions to 'lock out' the dense outside township world, temporarily as a non-policed and private sexual world. The toilet is never however entirely private (Magni & Reddy 2007). When Nokulunga and her sister open the toilet door they interrupt the privacy; invest in the moral production of sexuality, censuring sex; and report Sane to her mother for "naughty" sexual behaviour.

The South African township toilet, whether located in the school or in the communities, is often constructed as sexually contaminating with reports indicating its location as a coercive site creating increasing vulnerability for women and girls to sexual violence, abuse and rape (see Human Rights Watch 2001). Such evidence also suggests the failure of the South African government to provide proper housing creating vulnerabilities for women and girls. What is interesting about children's responses to AIDS and sex here is the varying means by which they negotiate the structural parameters defining their lives, framing sex as naughty and exciting, locating sex in the toilet not as coercive but also consensual—a private, sexualized space which they took delight in discussing as they did in its censure and regulation.

## AIDS: SEX AND RAPE

### Men as Vectors in the Spread of the Disease

Sexual coercion and male culpability however remained a powerful gaze upon children's responses to AIDS. Male violence against women and girls is prevalent in many settings and often the root of women's heightened vulnerability to AIDS. In South Africa violence, as noted by Posel (2005), is often seen as the "scandal of manhood" and both boys and girls lock into this scandal:

| | |
|---|---|
| DB: | Who rapes? |
| Scelo (b): | It's the fathers. |
| DB: | How? |
| Scelo (b): | They go to their girlfriends and sleep with them and get AIDS. |
| Nontobeko: | Sometimes they rape kids then go to another place and rape there again. |
| Nokulunga: | It's boys. |
| Nokulunga: | They go to the girls and rape them. |
| Zibuyile: | Boys give us AIDS. |
| DB: | How? |
| Zibuyile: | They go out with a girl and he has sex with her . . . |
| Thuso (b): | He rapes her! |
| Nhlanhla (b): | He rapes her. Then she gets it. Then he goes out with another one and she gets it too. |
| Thuso (b): | They ask a girl out and have sex with her and then dump her and go out with another one. |
| Nomusa: | Men, they rape kids. |
| Wendy: | It's men that spread this disease, because we heard from women how it started. I know its men, because usually they rape a girl, and go and keep changing and sharing this woman. And maybe she already has AIDS, and they go and rape other ones. |
| Pindile: | Men. They rape and rape and don't care. |
| Snikiwe: | It's men because they rape and rape they don't use condoms. |
| DB: | What is a condom? |
| Snikiwe: | It's a plastic object that protect you from getting AIDS and most people don't use it. |

Unlike the previous analyses, the discussion here is ominous, with men and boys especially being targeted as vectors in the spread of the disease. The engagement in violent and coercive sexual relations is often encouraged for "real men" (Mane & Aggleton 2001). Both boys and girls confirm the status of adult men at the apex of the age/gender hierarchy who feed on male entitlement to sex through violence heightening women's and girls' risk to disease (Wood & Jewkes 2001). The responses must be situated within discourses of violent gender and patriarchal relations and their structural location in the township. As Jewkes *et al.* (2006) report the very scale of sexual violence and rape in South Africa suggests that important aspects of South African society, if not legitimating, at least provide the space for these activities. Children know of such activity and they highlight its brutality: "they rape and rape and don't care." Such violence also instils and reproduces the fear of men and the lack of power of women and children in relation to men. Dominant narratives of blame for the spread of HIV are often placed on women (LeClerc-Madlala 2001) and whilst this is discussed in the next part of this section, here both boys and girls target adult men as the source of their vulnerability and who are blamed further for not wearing condoms in preventing AIDS. Situating their understandings of male power within the framework of a rampant heterosexual masculinity, the children are particularly scathing in their attack on men, highlighting as they do the highly unequal gender and age relations in sexual violations. Significantly, children are subjects speaking out about the politics of AIDS, albeit in an environment which constrains their freedoms.

## Girls Spread AIDS!

Children inhabited (as they contested) dominant narratives of blame framed around female sexuality. Women were regarded as 'reservoirs of infection' with problematic sexual practices and social behaviours:

| | |
|---|---|
| Sibusiso (b): | Girls spread AIDS. |
| DB: | How? |
| Sphamandla (b): | They sleep with a boy and then sleeps with another. |
| Andile (b): | It's males. |
| Hloniphani (b): | No, I'm saying that it's females. |
| DB: | Why? |
| Wendy: | No it's boys because they . . . sleep around and they keep infecting innocent people. |
| Sboniso (b): | I say women because they sleep around, they are prostitutes. |

The ongoing gendered permutations and contestations locate sexuality as a medium through which AIDS is represented. Contrary to the view that young African children cannot make sense of their sexuality (van Dyk 2008), the children here present as active participants rejecting, contesting and locking into gender scripts which try to position women as "prostitutes"—sleeping around, carriers of disease and stigmatized for deviant and promiscuous behaviour. Sboniso's claim positions men as passive recipients of the disease but is contested by Wendy, who frames women as "innocent". Andile is the only boy in the group who does not form part of the collective attack on women, but he does so in an atmosphere that attempts to confirm male hegemony.

From a young age boys are learning to reproduce gender inequalities, placing female sexuality under a male gaze:

| | |
|---|---|
| Hloniphani (b): | When a person is raped sometimes it's by force, and sometimes they ask for it. |
| DB: | How do they ask for it? |
| Hloniphani (b): | They show off their bodies. Some people wear G-strings and short skirts and tops, and when they bend boys see their G-string all the way. |
| DB: | And you? |
| Mthoko (b): | Sometimes it's by force, sometimes they cause it for themselves because they don't dress properly. |
| Nhlaka (b): | I'm saying males. |
| DB: | What do they do? |
| Nhlaka (b): | They rape women and they always that disease even more, because they sleep with females by force. |

Hloniphani begins the discussion by arguing that rape (and the consequence of disease) is caused by women who "ask for it", and this is confirmed by Mthoko, who says that women "cause it for themselves because they don't dress properly". Within local contexts, social and cultural relations between men and women are governed by a notion of respect that dictates appropriate practices in women's dress. Men are "forced" to rape women because they dare to breach this code, an argument confirmed by Moffet (2006). Showing off bodies and wearing G-strings, short skirts and tops are considered unacceptable and sufficiently subversive and threatening to Zulu cultural practices, compelling men to discipline them through sexual violence. Hloniphani asserts this view. Both sexual and physical violence against women form part of a repertoire of strategies of male control (Wood & Jewkes 2001) and feature strongly in the dominant social constructions of masculinity in South Africa. Seven- and eight-year-old boys are already inscribing within these normative boundaries and are punitive towards women who do not recognise their place in the gender hierarchy. Women who attempt to break out of cultural definitions of appropriate dress are punished. Risk of exposure to HIV is related to women who show their "G-strings" placing the responsibility for controlling men's sexual desires and rape on women and girls. When "boys see their G-strings all the way" results in an uncontrollable male desire, a discursive device to coerce girls into more conservative styles of dressing and behaviour and to remind them of the need to respect (inherently uncontrollable dangerous) men and boys (see Jewkes et al. 2006). There are consequences for violation of respect to men as recent South African media reports suggest. Taxi drivers and hawkers joined forces to teach an African woman a lesson in Johannesburg. Nwabisa Ngcukana, 25, was stripped and sexually assaulted for wearing a mini-skirt. In a township in Durban, KwaZulu-Natal, a woman was stripped naked by a gang of men and her house burned down for wearing trousers (*Mail & Guardian*

2008). The fear of men and the implications for younger girls' vulnerability is heightened, as the next section shows.

## Girls Fear Men

The fear of men was widespread in the focus group interviews, but it was girls in particular who felt most vulnerable to men and rape:

| | |
|---|---|
| Nomusa: | I always pray that I don't get it [AIDS]. |
| Wendy: | Yes, from school I go straight home. I talk to nobody. |
| DB: | Why? |
| Wendy: | Because I know that some people when they see children . . . they snatch kids and they get away. |
| Nomusa: | I will stay away from boys. |
| DB: | Why? |
| Nomusa: | They want to rape children. |
| DB: | Why do you think they do that to children? |
| Nomusa: | I know that from experience, because when we were walking home with my friends and this guy, he is a very old man, he came after us, he was running after us I don't know about my friends, but I fled home. One of them was nearly caught by this man. I know that he's not good. |
| DB: | Anele, you want to say something? |
| Anele: | Sometimes he buys us chocolate. |
| Hlengiwe: | We were a group of six and this same old guy came and bought us sweets. But we didn't eat them because our parents know about him, they said if anyone who gives us something we must throw it away, and we always throw it away. |

Propitious conditions prevail in townships increasing and creating high-risk situations for women and girls to sexual abuse and HIV. Contrary to the view that African children are helpless victims, the girls earlier spoke as active participants in articulating their vulnerability. They do not speak self-pityingly even if the social conditions that lead to their vulnerability and fear of men arouse pity. The accumulation of social violence, coupled with the social and cultural norms defining gender and age hierarchies, has produced a context in which girls' fear of men in the township is ascendant. This context is not of their own making, and even under these circumstances the girls creatively talk about the resources they use in protecting themselves ranging from praying, fleeing from bad men, going straight home, not talk-ing to anybody on the way from school, staying away from boys, rejecting the offer of sweets and, finally, obeying parents, as Hlengiwe asserts. Nego-tiating the circumstances of social violence and the lack of social capital, they talk about the resources they can muster in dealing with the threat of men—both actual and imagined. Their fear of men is situational, the effect of material, discursive and symbolic forces constraining opportunities and choices available to them. Whilst their strategies in dealing with their fear of men are admirable in negotiating the structural parameters defining their lives, they are certainly at higher risk to rape and HIV. As Craddock (2004) argues, young women and girls suffer disproportionately, sometimes experiencing rates of infection four to five times higher than boys in the same age group. As Craddock's research and others suggest, the ways in which poverty, gender and generational lines, as well as ongoing economic insecurities intersect might help to explain the embeddedness of social vulnerability to AIDS creating high risk situations for children especially young girls (see also Schoepf 2004).

## AIDS PREVENTION

On the issue of prevention, not only did the children have a great deal of knowledge of condoms, but they also tied prevention to sexual coercion and highly unequal gender inequalities:

| | |
|---|---|
| DB: | How will you protect yourself from AIDS? |
| Sipho (b): | I will use a condom. |
| Zanele: | I will just make sure that I stay at home after school hours. If a stranger tries to call me I will run away and call my mother. |
| Wendy: | I won't have sex. |
| Nomusa: | No, because we say no to sex then he still rapes you. |
| Patrick (b): | Don't go sleeping around with boys. |
| Nhlanhla (b): | Boys must sleep in the bed and the girls must sleep on the floor. |
| Wendy: | But what happens is that when the girl is asleep the boy sneaks into the bed and sleeps with the girl. |

"I will" or "I won't" are strong indicators of children's agency. As they assert their knowledge they creatively build on strategies to protect themselves. Such agency relates to potentially using a condom; staying at home after school; running from strangers; relying on mother's support, a strategy noted by Zanele; saying no to sex; and abstaining. Amidst the fear, children have their own strategies in place. Zanele relies on her mother for social support, drawing strength against the formidable construction of the masculinised stranger. Wider social tensions around the disease however resulting from material and discursive forces effectively constrain the opportunities and choices available to young children and potentially create conditions of vulnerability: "[W]e say no . . . then he still rapes." The social context of risk to sexual violence and HIV, their vulnerability to men and rape and the restriction to agency situates AIDS prevention strategies firmly within these complexities. Saying no is patent evidence that this strategy will not work in prevention unless the aggregate effects of sexual violence, unequal gender/age inequalities and the embeddedness of social vulnerability to AIDS are understood within local contexts.

The weight of HIV prevention as Wendy asserts is embedded within highly unequal gender inequalities and sexual violence and in a social context manufacturing such relations. As Schoepf (2004) argues, in much of Africa, economic and cultural factors circumscribe the ability of girls to refuse sex or to insist on condom use. The status of men in relation to the ability of young girls to say no, as Nomusa testifies, situates prevention within a dominating social system in which men have power particularly over young girls exacerbating vulnerability, reducing girls' ability to refuse sexual advances and reproducing male power and control. Safe sex, using a condom and saying no suggest that even at ages seven and eight, the children are able to understand prevention strategies. Young children have highly sophisticated knowledge of AIDS prevention. When children here demonstrate understanding of AIDS, sex, rape and condoms, they go against the commonly held view of incapacity and incompetence around health issues (Alderson 2007). Their acute sense of knowledge has developed through direct social and personal experience of communities affected and infected with HIV. Their agency is constrained through social and age inequalities in a context in which sexual violence and rape is pervasive. The problem of rape in South Africa as Wood and Jewkes (2001) show has to be understood within the context of the very substantial gender power inequalities that pervade South African society. Rape is a manifestation of male dominance over women, and as Jewkes *et al.* (2006) claim, rape is an assertion of that position. This tragedy embodies that of township life with its legacy of race, class and gender inequalities and the culture of AIDS. Seven- and eight-year-olds often marginalized in discussion around AIDS, gender, sexuality and prevention are already inscribing within these discourses; they know their vulnerability and speak up about it.

## CONCLUSION

Analysis rooted in the agency of young African children—rarely featuring in research and debates about AIDS—has an important role to play in replacing stereotypes with accounts that recognise the complex and contested processes through children engage with the disease. Their agency is negotiated within complex social processes involving not only sexual violence and highly unequal gender/age inequalities but also sexual expression. Those expressions are subsumed, however, under a regime of violence and fear catapulting men, albeit with contestation, as chief vectors in the spread of the disease and a source of girls' anxieties. The responses to male power, sexual violence and gender inequalities in the construction of AIDS are the effect or effects of material, symbolic and discursive forces constraining the opportunities available to them and creating patterns of vulnerability to the disease—especially for young girls (Jewkes & Morrell 2012). Rape and the fear of rape squeeze agency and are abetted by contemporary patterns of male power within extreme settings such as KwaDabeka.

In the last decade, emerging work on the study of gender, sexuality and AIDS in South Africa (Wood & Jewkes 2001; Hallman 2007; Harrison 2008; Jewkes & Morrell 2012) have correctly stressed the deep social roots of violence creating patterns of vulnerability and risk for women and girls. But so, too, must scholars begin to reassess how younger boys and girls—often peripheral in strategies around debate, research and prevention—give meaning to gender and sexuality in their account of the disease and their notions of risk. The African township has provided a critical vantage point to understand the negotiations around gender and sexuality, the gendered patterns of risk and the reproduction of the scandal of manhood, albeit with contestation. Empowering models of children's ability to navigate their social worlds and influence the environments in which they live (Parkes 2008) have been neglected in young children's account of AIDS. Young African girls are not waiting to be victims of AIDS; both boys and girls reject dominant forms of masculinity which create vulnerability, even as they reproduce ideas that women are reservoirs of infection. Male power is not monolithic, even though masculine power and violence have been tragically noted by children as creating patterns of vulnerability and fear. The flexibility of gender relations point to generating AIDS education that is responsive to young children's capacity to think sexually and to respond to gender/age relations that create patterns of vulnerabilities. Schools, teachers and parents do have a responsibility to address these concerns.

What can children do in these contexts? Clearly, young children have sophisticated knowledge of sex as pleasure and danger, as well as intimate knowledge of the disease and prevention: "we say no to sex then he still rapes you." Age inequalities, gender and sexual asymmetries of power combined with the social and cultural context of KwaDabeka are important to recognise in young children's anger towards men more generally rather than an essentialist picture of "bad men". Zulu cultural practices called *ukuhlonipha* are important in understanding the mediation and construction of knowledge around men. Carton (2001) refers to *ukuhlonipha* as customs of avoidance and deference that reflect generational/gendered divisions where men are at the apex of the age/gender hierarchy. In relation to older men, younger children (and girls in particular) remain more vulnerable to sexual abuse and rape (see Richter *et al.* 2004). As Nomusa and Wendy indicate, material/cultural constructions of gender relations create patterns of vulnerability especially for women and girls. Girls do speak out. They contest the dominant cultural norms that try to put them in their place even as they reproduce it, but their ability to choose and to assert themselves takes place in conditions not of their own making.

Any attempt to promote young people's right to knowledge about the disease and its relationship with gender and sexuality will stumble without parallel attempts to undo the constraints to children's agency in the broader context. Agency depends on the ability to exercise that agency in the context where both boys and girls are located. The exercise of children's agency is socially embedded. As Bhana's (2008) study shows, amongst a predominantly white context, seven- and eight-year-old children draw on contagion and power inequalities to reproduce racist constructions of the disease, but they also show empathy and care. Contextual specific research is important in the study of young children and HIV (Cobbett et al 2013).

Interventions that attempt to address gender equality in AIDS education without developing a context that fosters its operation are in danger of replicating the fear that girls feel and the sense of entitlement that young boys are already learning in the making of manhood. Given the burden of the complexity of gender and sexuality in creating patterns of vulnerability to and experience of AIDS within specific contexts, many scholars have argued for greater scrutiny of the effects of gender power inequalities and economic conditions when targeting interventions (see Schoepf 2004; Harrison 2008). Poverty, violence and pervasive gender inequality continue to make it difficult for women and girls to avoid unsafe sex. Young children know this even at ages seven and eight, and girls are rendered particularly vulnerable in their fear of men. There is need to address and challenge the combination of gender/age inequalities, social and economic depression, sexual violence and the cultural politics that maintain unequal hierarchies in order to understand more comprehensively what it will take to intervene effectively into children's vulnerability in the context of AIDS.

## REFERENCES

Alderson, P. (2007)' Competent Children? Minors' Consent to Health Care Treatment and Research'. *Social Science and Medicine*, 65: 2272–2283.

Bhana, D. (2008). 'Beyond Stigma? Young Children's Responses to AIDS'. *Culture Health and Sexuality*, 10(7): 725–738.

Bhana, D. & Epstein, D. (2007) ' "I Don't Want to Catch It" Boys, Girls and Sexualities in an HIV Environment'. *Gender and Education*, 19(1): 109–125.

Blaise, M. (2010) 'Kiss and Tell: Gendered Narratives and Childhood Sexuality'. *Australasian Journal of Early Childhood*, 35 (1): 1–9.

Carton, B. (2001). 'Locusts Fall From the Sky: Manhood and Migrancy in Kwa-Zulu', in R. Morrell (ed) *Changing Men in South Africa* (pp. 1–64). Pietermaritzburg: University of Natal Press.

Chong, E., Hallman, K. & Brady, M. (2006). *Investing When it Counts*. New York: UNFPA and Population Council.

Cobbett, M., McLaughlin, C. & Kiragu, S. (2013) 'Creating "Participatory Spaces": Involving Children in Planning Sex Education Lessons in Kenya, Ghana and Swaziland'. *Sex Education*, 13(1): S70–S83.

Craddock, S. (2004) 'Beyond Epidemiology: Locating AIDS in Africa', in E. Kalipeni, E. Craddock, S. Oppong & J. Ghosh (eds), *AIDS in Africa Beyond Epidemiology* (pp. 1–10). Oxford: Blackwell Publishing.

Delius, P. & Glaser, C. (2005) 'Sex, Disease and Stigma in South Africa: Historical Perspectives'. *African Journal of AIDS Research*, 4(1): 29–36.

Delius, P. & Glaser, C. (2002) 'Sexual Socialization in South Africa: A Historical Perspective'. *African Studies*, 61: 27–54.

Hallman, K. (2007) 'Sexuality, Reproductive Health and HIV/AIDS: Non-Consensual Sex, School Enrolment and Educational Outcomes in South Africa'. *Africa Insight*, 37(3): 454–472.

Harrison, A. (2008). 'Hidden Love: Sexual Ideologies and Relationship Ideals Among Rural South African Adolescents in the Context of HIV/AIDS'. *Culture Health and Sexuality*, 10(2): 175–189.

Human Rights Watch. (2001). *Scared at School: Sexual Violence Against Girls in South African Schools*. New York: Human Rights Watch.

Jewkes, R. & Abrahams, N. (2002) 'The Epidemiology of Rape and Sexual Coercion in South Africa: An Overview'. *Social Science and Medicine*, 55: 1231–1244.

Jewkes, R., Dunkle, K., Koss, M. P., Levin, J. B., Ndunae, M., Jamaa, N. & Sikweyiya, Y. (2006) 'Rape Perpetration by Young, Rural South African Men: Prevalence, Patterns and Risk Factors'. *Social Science & Medicine*, 63: 2949–2961.

Jewkes, R., Flood, M. & Lang, J. (2014) 'From Work With Men and Boys to Changes of Social Norms and Reduction of Inequities in Gender Relations: A Conceptual Shift in Prevention of Violence Against Women and Girls'. *The Lancet*, 385 (9977) : 1580-1589.

Jewkes, R., Levin, J., Mbananga, N. & Bradshaw, D. (2002) 'Rape of Girls in South Africa'. *Lancet*, 359: 319–320.

Jewkes, R. & Morrell, R. (2012) 'Sexuality and the Limits of Agency Among South African Teenage Women: Theorising Femininities and Their Connections to HIV Risk Practises'. *Social Science & Medicine*, 74(11): 1729–1737.

Jewkes, R., Penn-Kekana, L. & Rose-Junius, H. (2005). ' "If They Rape Me, I Can't Blame Them": Reflections on Gender in the Social Context of Child Rape in South Africa and Namibia'. *Social Science & Medicine*, 61: 1809–1820

Le Clerc Madlala, S. (2001). 'Virginity Testing: Managing Sexuality in a Maturing HIV/AIDS Epidemic'. *Medical Anthropology Quarterly*, 15(4): 533–553.

Mager, A. (1999). *Gender and the Making of a South African Bantustan: A Social History of the Ciskei 1945–1959*. Portsmouth, NH: Heinemann.

Magni, S. & Reddy, V. (2007). 'Performative Queer Identities: Masculinities and Public Bathroom Usage'. *Sexualities*, 10(2): 229–242.

*Mail & Guardian* (19 February 2008). 'Outrage Over Attack on Miniskirt-Wearing Woman'. http://www.mg.co.za/article/2008-02-19-outrage-over-attack-on-miniskirt wearing-woman, accessed 10 July 2008.

Mane, P. & Aggleton, P. (2001). 'Gender and HIV/AIDS: What Do Men Have to Do With it?' *Current Sociology*, 49: 23–38.

Moffett, H. (2006). ' "These Women, They Force Us to Rape Them": Rape as narrative of Social Control in Post-Apartheid South Africa'. *Journal of Southern African Studies*, 32(1): 131–144.

Nayak, A. & Kehily. M. J. (2001). ' "Learning to Laugh": A Study of Schoolboy Humour in the English Secondary School', in W. Martino & B. Meyenn (eds), *What About The Boys? Issues of Masculinity in Schools* (pp. 110–124). Buckingham: Open University Press.

Parkes, J. (2008). 'The Multiple Meanings of Violence. Children's Talk About Life in a South African Neighbourhood'. *Childhood*, 14(4): 401–414.

Posel, D. (2005). 'The Scandal of Manhood: "Baby Rape" and the Politicization of Sexual Violence in Post-Apartheid South Africa'. *Culture Health and Sexuality*, 7 (3): 239–252.

Reddy, V. (2004). 'Sexuality in Africa: some trends, transgressions and tirades'. *Agenda*, 62: 3–11.

Renold, E. (2005). *Girls, Boys and Junior Sexualities: Exploring Children's Gender and Sexual Relations in the Primary School*. London: RoutledgeFalmer.

Richter, L., Dawes, A. & Higson-Smith, C. (eds). (2004) *Sexual Abuse of Young Children in Southern Africa*. Cape Town: HSRC Press.

Robinson, S. (2013) 'Regulating the Race: Aboriginal Children in Private European Homes in Colonial Australia'. *Journal of Australian Studies*, 37(3): 302–315.

Schoepf, B.G. (2004). 'AIDS in Africa: Structure, Agency and Risk', in E. Kalipeni, E. Craddock, S. Oppong & J. Ghosh (eds) *AIDS in Africa Beyond Epidemiology* (pp. 121–133). Oxford: Blackwell Publishing.

Thorne, B. (1993). *Gender Play: Girls and Boys in School*. New Brunswick, NJ: Rutgers University Press.

van Dyk, A. (2008). 'Perspectives of South African School Children on HIV/AIDS, and the Implications for Education Programmes'. *African Journal of AIDS Research*, 7(1): 79–93.

Wood, K. & Jewkes, R. (2001) ' "Dangerous" Love: Reflections on Violence Among Xhosa Township Youth', in R. Morrell (ed), *Changing Men in Southern Africa* (pp 317–336). Pietermaritzburg: University of Natal Press.

Wood, K., Lambert, H. & Jewkes, R. (2007). 'Showing Roughness in a Beautiful Way'. *Medical Anthropology Quarterly*, 21 (3): 277–300.

# 5 AIDS and Age
## Children Negotiating and Resisting Sexual Knowledge

DB:      But should teachers talk about it [AIDS]?
Daniel:  Good question. I don't know.

—Conversation at Bullwood

Boys and girls manoeuvre the social, economic, and cultural context of AIDS in South Africa and their knowledge is embedded within and contingent upon these social processes. Chapters 2, 3 and 4 have illustrated the complex mesh through which children weave through the social context of AIDS and tear apart discourses of childhood innocence. But children can also uphold innocence. Childhood innocence represents a cluster of discourses and practices surrounding sex and sexuality, power and authority. I was struck by the unpredictable ways in which sex appeared and disappeared. The children's discussion was haphazard, moving from contagion, blood, germs, dirt to sex as they invoked gender, sexuality, race and class inequalities and challenged, promoted and rejected childhood innocence (James *et al.* 1998). I began this chapter with seven-year-old Daniel at Bullwood, who talked extensively about the sexual route of AIDS and yet was not sure whether adult teachers should engage children about the disease.

When children were asked, "Should your teachers/parents talk to you about AIDS?" they reflected, negotiated and resisted sexual knowledge. Like Daniel, children negotiate hegemonic discourses of childhood innocence. In this chapter, I consider children's tactical strategies through which the sexual content of AIDS-related knowledge is mediated, negotiated and resisted. Having sexual knowledge of the disease, or too much of it can stain childhood innocence but having and expressing sexual knowledge and desires can also produce excitement, laughter, shame, embarrassment and pleasure. Adults would like children to be innocent (Kehily 2004), and children can contribute to that idealisation, in order to be seen as the ideal child. They also break it down, adjust it and contest these definitions. The boundaries between knowing about sex and AIDS and not knowing are very slippery, creating many conditions for transgression. Childhood innocence is thus not passively accepted. Children do negotiate what it means to have sexual knowledge within an overall regulatory environment where innocence is hegemonic. Children may not be passive, but they, too, conspire in presenting the glorification of childhood innocence (Silin 1995).

In this chapter, I illustrate how children regularly move in out and of the discourse of childhood innocence and in and out of more adult discourses of sexuality (Renold 2005). They are highly alert to discourses which function to position childhood innocence as normative, and they regularly take up the position as 'innocent', needing protection from dangerous sexual knowledge, germs and health problems just as they regularly give meaning to the sexual route of transmission. As Silin (1995: 171) argues, when it comes to children's knowledge of sex they "tacitly accede to the mutual presence that assures their place in the work as the unknowing child the thus display their own command of the social system enabling adults to play the familiar part of the knowledgeable without embarrassment". Children are active in this process of strategising about what is appropriate to learn about, from the adult perspective. Whilst children in both schools made very explicit connections between sex and AIDS, it was quickly accompanied, as this chapter shows, by anxieties related to sexual knowledge, and children often said, "Please, don't tell the teacher." Children give command to their place within the social system as they hide, deny and silence sex in AIDS-related knowledge enabling childhood to function within familiar relations of power as they strengthen the social fabric of innocence. Children's anxieties are reflective of adult concerns of sexuality (Thorne 1993). Children do know the benefits of their place as innocent and young. They understand the taboos regarding too much of sexual knowledge at age seven and eight. From an adult perspective, being 'too young' provides evidence of children's incomplete constructions as adults, unprotesting and without agency. Children know this as a powerful marker of adult–child relations and work on this, not passively but actively commanding their place as the mockery of childhood innocence is revealed. Children simultaneously deny and acknowledge sexuality as key to HIV transmission. As children work on what to know sexually, they validate adult constructions of children's assumed ignorance and innocence as they validate their agency.

## RESISTING SEXUAL KNOWLEDGE: TOO YOUNG TO KNOW

In this part of the chapter I illustrate how children regulate their sexual knowledge of the disease by upholding childhood innocence and invoking age gradation and levels of maturity underpinned by developmental theory to cast doubt on their knowledge of sex and present the ideal version of childhood. As I have argued, the sexual knowledge of AIDS appears together with other aspects of the disease, including contagion.

**Bullwood**

| | |
|---|---|
| Andrew: | I also wanna know how you can get AIDS 'cause in the Oreo packs there's these stickers . . . I watched it on TV . . . one person stuck it on them and underneath . . . there's AIDS underneath them and it soaks into the holes in your skin . . . |
| Kayla: | . . . [J]a, like if you are not married and like you have sex or something like that. . . people say that you get AIDS if you like have sex and you're not married. |
| Daniel: | Like say a girl has AIDS and like you, you're a boy and you go have sex with her then you can get AIDS. And say you quickly run to the doctor and if the doctor says that you got HIV positive then you got AIDS and if they say you are HIV negative that means you did not get AIDS. |
| Cody: | Hey, that's age restricted . . . |
| DB: | Why? |
| Cody: | . . .'[C]ause we're too young to understand it. |

Cody draws attention to regulatory forces that demarcate what knowledge is appropriate for children (MacNaughton 2000). Kayla's version of AIDS conflicts with Andrew, who wants to know about how the disease is spread and draws on Oreo stickers as a route of transmission invoking contagion. Kayla presents sex within marriage as a safety locus and sex outside of marriage as risk for the disease. Sex is safe in marriage, and in contrast, sex outside of marriage is contaminated by disease. Cody's response to the explicit mention of sex is to regulate the conversation by drawing on age-restricted knowledge. The conversation shifts to age-restricted movies because children's heightened awareness of sexual surveillance is evident as resistance:

| | |
|---|---|
| Cody: | And also they have got movies that have age restrictions on that. You're not allowed to watch them 'cause it's not good for children to watch them, they have got an age like 16. |
| Andrew: | It's because if you put the age restriction up, it tells you what type of movie it is. It tells you 'L'—that's for language, and 'S' is for sex and, er, . . . |
| Cody: | And PG is for parental guidance. But if the movie says 13 then there's no under-13. |
| Andrew: | But the *Bourne Identity*—that's fine. |
| Cody: | *Ja*, but PG [parental guidance], like just PG means that your mom has to check. |
| Andrew: | I know. I'm not allowed to watch any movies like *Carte Blanche*. |
| DB: | Why? |

Andrew:   Oh, only some . . . *Ja*, some of them aren't nice.

Cody:   I'm also allowed to watch *Carte Blanche* only sometimes and then I take long to eat. [Giggling] . . . Every Sunday I eat slowly in the lounge. . . so my mom's like, "hurry up, hurry up" . . . And I just keep eating slow.

Childhood sexuality, as Foucault (1978), notes is under surveillance by a watch crew that includes parents. Children are aware of the heightened attention to age appropriate knowledge and censorship (Robinson 2013). Authority and power vested in adults to dictate the terms of appropriate knowledge and age restriction is key. The children refer to *Carte Blanche*, a local documentary often providing graphic details of South African life. Sometimes viewers are alerted to the sensitive nature of its content, which makes it unsuitable for children, but as Cody suggests, even age-restricted programming is open to resistance. Childhood innocence whilst powerful is contested.

Children often referred to delaying sexual knowledge, to later grades and ages as they upheld childhood innocence with some referring to high schools and grade 5 as more appropriate for AIDS education. This was despite having sexual knowledge of the disease.

## Bullwood

Kirsty:   I think it's because we're too young to know. I don't know but I think we are too young to know.

DB:   Too young. What age should we talk about it?

Tiffany:   I don't know. We are all eight in our class. Some of them are seven. I don't think that our teacher is gonna talk about it.

Kirsty:   Maybe after grade five, I think that we should be learning about it . . .

Zak:   We probably should be doing it in high school when we [are] doing projects . . . In high school my mum says all high school children have to get a mouse and cut it open and see it's heart and if it's not dead they gonna do a big test . . . Stinks!

Children regulate as they are regulated by the hegemonic discourse of childhood innocence. Children's reluctance to engage formally with AIDS reveals the ways in which normative meanings around age, young and innocence are being deployed for the collective production and reproduction of childhood innocence. Children are extremely responsive to childhood discursive cues. A uniformity of meaning around childhood innocence was evident in both schools where children also drew on the affective dynamics of childhood sexuality and produced a collective meaning around not knowing.

The attempt to erase sexuality or delay it as an accomplishment of maturity can be seen as an attempt by the children to adopt adult positions and to project innocence.

## KwaDabeka

Andile:   They don't make us feel good.
DB:       Why?
Andile:   We don't like talking about them.
DB:       Why?
Andile:   We don't like to be taught bad things. We're still young.

By engaging with oppositional rhetoric children displace sexuality from their lives and seek to eliminate sex and AIDS education. By associating it with a specific set of meanings, Andile's words situate sex within the negative, inciting the need for protection from all things sexual. The transcripts show how, through the children's deploying adult versions of childhood sexuality, the recourse to sexual innocence, developmental outcomes and the displacement of agency combine to function as part of a strategic tactic in regulating and maintaining the myth of innocence. In other words, children at both schools are moving into a discourse of innocence and are controlling and eliminating sexual discussion that best allows for the protection of young children. Sex is associated with bad things, as being evil and salacious. The oppositional rhetoric operates as part of the social control of sexuality, and this serves an important task in the production of childhood innocence.

## Bullwood

DB:       And you should we talk about AIDS?
Tanya:    No 'cause we normally do work. Maybe when we get to high school we might talk about it.
DB:       Now tell me why only in high school?
Tanya:    That's when they teach you a lot of things and that's when you understand and that's when you are bigger.
DB:       Don't you understand anything now?
Tanya:    Just a little bit.

It must be noted here that Tanya's response illustrated detailed knowledge of sex and AIDS. She was able to articulate with confidence knowledge of sex and HIV transmission, but she was also inserting within a discourse which positioned her as a child and through which she, too, positioned herself displacing sex and AIDS education to "high school". The trouble and the risks in knowing the relationship between AIDS and sex are clear as indicated in the following excerpt.

## Bullwood

Karen:   *Ja*, . . . I don't know about that stuff. My mum told me that I am not supposed to know about it. We might get into trouble.
DB:   Why?
Karen:   I don't know.
DB:   How would you get into trouble?
Dianne:   You can get into trouble 'cause you aren't supposed to talk about AIDS in the class.
DB:   I see many of you talking in the classroom.
Dianne:   *Ja*, but you get shouted at.
DB:   Why?
Dianne:   We get shouted at 'cause we are talking.

Having sexual knowledge and making the connection with AIDS are thus troubling for young children who are "not supposed to know about it" because this knowledge is regulated by adult parents and teachers. Whilst young children in this study were thoughtful strategists about what they said in response to sexual knowledge and AIDS, they, too, are highly alert to the risks involved in knowing sexually. They know that age-specific determinants deem what is acceptable, although they certainly do not simply reproduce this version of the child. They realise though that their age and sexuality are under the adult gaze and are policed by the boundaries of innocence as they, too, police themselves.

## KwaDabeka

DB:   Why don't you talk about AIDS in the classroom?
Anton:   Because *tisha* [teacher] will beat me up.
DB:   Why?
Anton:   I might say something wrong.
Abigail:   . . . [L]ike they sleep . . . like if a boy is sleeping and girl sleeping with him together . . . sleeping together . . . I mean the boy and girl they sleep together and you have AIDS and the boy doesn't wear a condom . . . like that, that's wrong . . .

Demonstrating the connection among sex and AIDS and sleeping together and condoms are clearly indications of the extent to which some children do know of sex and AIDS. In the regulation of sexuality, Anton shows that having knowledge of sex and AIDS is not only restricted by discourses of childhood innocence but through corporal punishment, particular to KwaDabeka. Whilst corporal punishment has been banned in many schools, particularly in African township schools, the practice continues (Department of Education 1996). Talking about sex and AIDS was thus dangerous and harmful for children at the school with punitive consequences.

## KwaDabeka

| | |
|---|---|
| DB: | In class, do you about talk about AIDS? |
| Siya: | We are still young . . . we can't talk about AIDS. |
| Asante: | No. |
| DB: | Why? |
| Asante: | We'll get smacked . . . by the *tisha* [teacher]. |
| DB: | Why? |
| Siya: | Because it's older people's stuff. |
| DB: | Is it okay for the teachers to talk to you about HIV/AIDS? |
| Speshle: | No. |
| DB: | Why is that? |
| Speshle: | It's not right. |

When young children were asked whether they should talk about HIV/AIDS in the classroom, the responses were overwhelming "No", "It wouldn't be right", "Sex is not to be discussed by small children":

| | |
|---|---|
| DB: | Are we supposed to talk about AIDS? |
| Nkanyiso: | No. |
| DB: | Why? |
| Nkanyiso: | It doesn't make us feel good. |
| DB: | Why? |
| Thabiso: | We don't like talking about them. |
| DB: | Why? |
| Mlungisi: | We don't like to be taught bad things. |
| Silindile: | It's not right. |
| DB: | Why? |
| Mlungisi: | We are going to do it too. |
| DB: | You'll do it? |
| Silindile: | Maybe a girl says to a boy, "Come and have sex with me". |
| Nkanyiso: | We'll get smacked . . . by the teachers. |
| DB: | Why? |
| Silindile: | Because it's old people's stuff. |

By resisting the right to know about HIV/AIDS and about sex, the children were drawing on discourses of childhood innocence despite the richness of their knowing. These contradictions show very clearly the constant struggle that young children have to endure in trying to present themselves as the ideal child. The deployment of childhood innocence is a strategic tool in the manufacture of the adult's version of childhood. To adopt the position of adult is to allow childhood innocence to flourish and to mark out hierarchies—those who assert the right to know suffer the effects of being excluded from the mythical (but powerful) version of childhood. Discredited notions that children who know about sex do sex are also resurrected by Silindile, working to validate adult concerns about sexuality and young children. The rejection of the right to know and the negotiation around knowing is framed not only by dominant adult perceptions of childhood sexuality but also by the concrete knowledge that they will be "smacked". In South Africa corporal punishment has been banned since 1996, but its practice has not been completely eliminated, as suggested by the children themselves. Corporal punishment thus induces fear and limits and represses their sexual voices.

The tragedy of corporal punishment in the regulation of children's knowledge of AIDS and sex embodies the experiences at KwaDabeka. How much children know of the disease is situated within the common and general regulation of being too young to know but has local effects, including being "smacked". Yet, the contradictions were clear:

| | |
|---|---|
| DB: | It's not right! Why? |
| Asante: | We are going to do that too . . . maybe a girl says to a boy, "Come and have sex with me". |
| Sifiso: | Also it doesn't make us feel good . . . |
| Samantha: | And the boys will laugh . . . They [the boys] will know what the teacher is talking about . . . |
| Amanda: | A boy calls a girl and she comes to talk and then he says let's go and have sex . . . |
| DB: | What is sex? |
| Asante: | It's being naughty . . . You go to the toilet and you do naughty things. |
| Amanda: | A boy puts his *pipi* [penis] inside a girl . . . When a boy calls a girl then they go to the toilet together. Then they go to the toilet to talk. Usually they whisper so that none can hear them. |

Contradicting the myth that sexual knowledge is inappropriate for young children, the discussion again confirms their intimate knowledge of AIDS and sex. The contradictory accounts suggest that children were simultaneously powerful in asserting and resisting sexual knowledge. Children thus have a strategic toolkit of resources in the management of their sexuality, and this constant shift from proclaiming childhood innocence to transgressing it is suggestive of the ways in which young children see the association with sexuality as problematic. These contradictions show the struggle that young children have in trying to present themselves as the ideal child. The deployment of childhood innocence is a strategic tool in the manufacture of the adult's version of childhood and children too fuel that version as they tear it down.

Asante argues that discussion of sex will increase the likelihood of having sex (Irvine 2002). By silencing it formally (even as they vocally talk about it), it is assumed that sex will be deferred. Sex is also situated with feelings of discomfort and is constructed as naughty. Regulation of childhood sexual knowledge was thus achieved though efforts to silence the sexual connection with AIDS, putting sex into the domain of discomfort whilst simultaneously transgressing notions of childhood innocence with intimate reference to sexual knowledge and what actually happens when boys talk to girls in the toilet. The discomfort about sexual knowledge not only functions to set children and sexuality as oppositional but also to police each other in producing a combined version of childhood, that of innocence. To speak in support of sexual knowledge and AIDS education was also to risk the presentation of the idealised child and the risk of being beaten by the *tisha*.

Sex, as children at KwaDabeka have already learnt, happens in private spaces and is situated within private whispers and in the toilet. In the context of massive poverty and one-bedroom shacks their knowledge of AIDS reflects their understanding of sex resulting from material and social processes elucidating not only the tragedy of corporal punishment but also the uneven deployment of structural constraints with the consequence that the only space for sex and intimacy, for the children in KwaDabeka, is the toilet. Clearly children here illustrate how their knowledge of AIDS imbricates with sexual and social dynamics at the micro level at KwaDabeka and the toilet.

## Bullwood

> Carla:   I would go to an AIDS school to learn about AIDS and stuff. Like if someone comes from a[n] AIDS school and they know about AIDS, I would tell them to tell me like everything about AIDS. I would not feel so shy in front of all the people but the AIDS school actually knows more about AIDS than we know and like Mrs Sing would not feel so safe and maybe she would not tell you 'caue your mother and father don't want you to know about AIDS and stuff. I don't think that Mrs Sing would want to tell anyone about AIDS 'cause it's not really right and she is not the AIDS teacher. She is just a normal teacher teaching you to read and write and the AIDS school your mother and father are putting you there so that you can learn about AIDS . . .

At Bullwood, Carla displaces AIDS from the official 'normal' duty of school with a normal teacher doing official schoolwork, which is reading and writing. Again, like the previous examples Carla had a great deal to say about boys and boyfriends and girlfriends, including having intimate knowledge of sex and AIDS. Yet contradictorily and strategically she positions herself on the side of official discourse displacing knowledge of sex and AIDS to an "AIDS school", where she will not feel "shy in front of all the people". Feelings of shyness, embarrassment and humiliation in talking sexually, and linking AIDS to sex was pervasive in children's understandings and regulation of knowledge (Irvine 2002). She also places herself in the position of the teacher noting that Mrs Sing will not feel comfortable not only because it was "not really right" but also because of parental fears and regulations. School, however, becomes a place to read and write. You can learn about AIDS and sex in the AIDS school if you have the permission of your parents. But parents are not the best allies when dealing with sex education:

> DB:      Do teachers talk about it?
> Damian:  No, because we got more important work to do.
> DB:      Like what?
> Damian:  Like maths and spelling.

Ideas about the right to know about AIDS are socially patterned and regulated. At Bullwood, maths and spelling are seen to be of greater significance a point that Damian agrees with. Bhana *et al.* (2006) have argued that the broader social landscape has shaped the work of school in relation to AIDS education where middle-class white schools are not in the forefront of dealing with it.

## Bullwood

> Danie:   Well my parents don't normally talk about AIDS.
> Ashley:  I too know about it . . . you see some people like some people on TV and those people have sex with some other people and they don't have a test and then they won't know that they got AIDS.
> DB:      And you Trent?
> Trent:   I don't know.
> DB:      Do your parents talk to you? Do you think that they should?
> Sara:    No, no. I don't know.
> Trent:   They don't talk about it so I won't talk about it.
> DB:      Okay . . . so you think that they should.
> Sara:    Well if they want to, they can.
> DB:      So they don't talk about it with you? Do you think that they should?
> Sara:    Well if they want to they can, but I think that if we want to know we should say, "Mum can you please talk to me about AIDS?" And like they say, "No it's not your age" and you must not talk about it if you are not allowed to talk about it, and if they say yes, then you can talk about it and AIDS.

In the context of knowledge of AIDS, sex and testing, as earlier, Ashley notes, is the recognition that parents regulate childhood sexuality and knowledge of what is appropriate. Even as Trent, too, knows of the association the restriction to sexual knowledge demonstrates how children are active in the process of regulating their sexual knowledge within adult parent constraints. Equally important, however, is the way in which Sara accords children with the right to know and ask. It is not simply a matter of silence and regulation, but Sara's testimony points so powerfully to children's expression of interest and curiosity and the right to assert agency, even as the power to knowledge in the final analysis is determined by the parent and even as children silently and secretly know.

However, children are not just waiting for adult instruction. They suggest ways in which their agency and right to knowledge can be facilitated by approaching adults.

## Bullwood

This part of the chapter picks up on the contradictions between Gugu's and Thobeka's desire to preserve the adult view of themselves as innocent children and their stark descriptions of sex:

| | |
|---|---|
| Gugu: | Please don't say anything to Mrs Sing. Please, please, please. |
| DB: | No, no, no. This tape's for me only. It's not going to be used for anything else. So do you think we should talk about this stuff? |
| Gugu: | No, 'cause I think it's not a good education to learn about it 'cause we're too young. |
| Thobeka: | So, so young. |
| DB: | If you're young why can't you know about it? |
| Gugu: | It's not a very good education. |
| Thobeka: | It's not for us. It's for big people. Its not our, what's that word . . . business. It's not our business. Children shouldn't know about that . . . |
| DB: | But do you know about that? |
| Thobeka: | Yes, 'cause I watch *Takalani*. And Kimmi has AIDS. Kimmi's mom has AIDS and Kimmi was born with AIDS. *Ja*. Yes I have been learning from *Takalani* every day. |
| DB: | So they're talking to kids about AIDS. So should the school talk about AIDS to kids?' |
| Gugu: | Noooo! |
| DB: | But they're talking to you about AIDS on *Takalani Sesame*. |
| Thobeka: | 'Cause we'll get shy. |
| DB: | What will embarrass you or what will you feel shy about? |
| Thobeka: | How to sleep with [a] girl! |
| Gugu: | On TV they say whenever you have sex you must always wear a condom. |
| Thobeka: | Because if we talk about this in the class the teachers will send letters to my parents and then when my mom finds |

out about this my mom will shout at me, especially my dad. And, um, I know we mustn't talk about AIDS because it's disgusting and maybe everyone will run away.

Gugu:    When we talk about it the teachers are going to send a letter to our parents and then we're gonna get suspended and we have to go to another school.

DB:    And what makes you shy?

Gugu:    'Cause, he sticks his penis in the girls vagina that's the part I'm shy about.

DB:    Why does it make you feel shy?

Gugu:    It just does.

Drawing on discourses of childhood innocence, the girls attempt to work around their sexual knowledge in strategic ways. "Don't say anything to the teacher" reminds us that the teacher as adult is a highly regulatory force and children are aware of the illicitness of the conversation. "It's not our business" worked really well as the girls tried to negotiate their innocence and insert themselves within discourses which prohibit the idea of the child as agent. While the girls understood that AIDS and sex are intimately connected, in this conversation they expressed horror. The use of the word *disgusting* was a further attempt to show why children should be saved and protected from such knowledge—a very adult-like position. These contradictions show very clearly the struggle that young children face in trying to present themselves as the ideal child and how emotions are deployed in the construction of sexuality from pleasure and desire to disgust and contempt. The girls not only displayed sexuality and knew explicit sexual details but also attempted to hide this knowledge for fear of being punished. The core concern here is that excessive sexual knowledge is dangerous because it suggests the erosion of innocence. However, it also suggests the passion for ignorance in the education of children (Silin 1995; Tobin 1997): "Ignorance in children is equated with innocence, then precocious sexual knowledge suggests defilement and culpability" (Tobin 1997: 138). The fear of being suspended from school takes on different proportions for these girls, for economic reasons, because their schooling is subsidised and because of the censure they might face from their parents, particularly their fathers. In the following transcript, too, the children articulated the connection between AIDS and sex, but when asked whether they should talk about AIDS in the classroom there was a great deal of contestation, deliberation and resistance:

Rachel:    No, 'cause we are too young to understand it.

Kate:    I think that when you are about 16, I think.

DB:    Tam, should we learn about AIDS?

Tam:    I don't think so.

DB:    You don't? James what do you think, should we learn about AIDS?

| | |
|---|---|
| James: | Oh my God! Err, No. |
| DB: | Why Not? |
| James: | 'Cause we're too young. I think that when we are about 15, we should learn about it. [Laughing] |
| DB: | Now tell me what do you mean too young . . .? |
| James: | Errr . . . we won't understand. |
| Grant: | *Ja*, . . . we won't understand all that stuff about life. |
| DB: | About the germs? |
| Grant: | I know about the germs 'cause I'm learning about this thing on the computer. It's called the Clue Finder Adventure Tracks. You learn about all kinds of germs and why you must not get them. |
| Rachel: | Because we won't understand and we won't really know. |
| Tam: | And because mostly if you wanna learn about AIDS you have to watch . . . like things about AIDS but most ones are age restricted. |
| DB: | Do you think that they should be age restricted? |
| All: | No. [Chorus] |
| DB: | So should you not be talking about that in class? |
| All: | No. [Chorus] |
| James: | When you are older you can talk about it . . . also there's whole lot of big words in the germs like . . . like . . . HIV. |
| DB: | What's HIV? |
| Kate: | My mum said that . . . I asked her about it. She said that there's a special kind of a relationship between a man and a woman. The kind . . . [Laughing] |
| DB: | Do you think that we should be talking about AIDS and stuff like that in the classroom? |
| Tam: | Not really, no. We might get into trouble. |
| DB: | How would you get into trouble? |
| Tam | I don't know. |
| DB: | You can get into trouble 'cause you aren't supposed to talk about AIDS in the class. |
| Kate: | You are not allowed to talk in the class. |
| DB: | I see many of you talking in the classroom. |
| Kate: | *Ja*, but you get shouted at. |
| DB: | Shouted at? Why? 'Cause you aren't supposed to talk about what? |
| Tam: | We get shouted at 'cause we're talking. |

Children are often seen as being too young to be discussing issues that pertain to their sexuality and are silenced by adults. In the transcript above, the boys and girls demonstrated their struggles, anxieties and powers as they individually and collectively made sense of their sexual identities. While the children made clear connections between sexuality and HIV/AIDS, when asked whether they should talk about AIDS in the more public space of the classroom, they drew on familiar notions of childhood innocence. The transcript shows how, by deploying adult versions of childhood sexuality, the recourse to sexual innocence, stages of development, being without knowledge and a whole lot of big words work together as part of a strategic tactic in regulating and maintaining the myth of sexual innocence. Being "too young", as suggested by Rachel and James, provides evidence of children's incomplete constructions as adults, unprotesting and without agency. Within this developmental notion of maturity young children are seen as de-gendered, asexual and without sexual knowledge. "We don't understand germs", "All that stuff about life" and "We won't know" function strategically to give meaning to development outcomes and validate adult constructions of young children's assumed ignorance and innocence. While discourses of denial (despite earlier assertions and reference to the special relationship) and delay were being shored up, the children were imagining having sexual knowledge at the age of 15 or 16. The attempt to erase sexuality or delay it as an accomplishment of maturity can be seen as an attempt by the children to adopt adult positions and to project innocence.

But such strategies were not uninterrupted—James referred to his computer providing knowledge of germs and why knowing about germs can prevent disease; the group was highly vocal in their disapproval of age-restricted information, suggesting that they did not want to be policed and under surveillance, but, at the same time, they were governing and managing their sexual knowledge by actions that policed the boundaries of a pure childhood. The capacious ways in which young children make meaning of their rights to knowledge of AIDS and sexuality is evident in the transcript and they did so by navigating and resisting the realm of childhood sexuality. The contradictory accounts in the interviews suggest that both boys and girls were simultaneously powerful in asserting their rights and resisting their freedoms. Children thus have a strategic toolkit of resources in the management of their sexuality more broadly (Renold 2005). This constant shift from knowing to resisting is suggestive of the ways in which young children see the association with sexuality as problematic. These contradictions again show the struggle that young children have in trying to present themselves as the ideal child.

## AIDS, GENDER, SEX, SEXUALITY AND SHAME

AIDS invokes the sexual and the sexual produces ambiguity and contradictions of meaning including embarrassment, laughter, humour and shame (Banas *et al.* 2011; Barnes 2012; Allen 2014). Whilst many children were able to articulate with confidence the sexual transmission of HIV, they did so in ways that not only expressed their agency debunking the myth of childhood innocence but also inserted contradictorily within discourses of shame and embarrassment (Irvine 2002; Blaise 2005). Childhood sexuality is enacted and consolidated within a realm where sex produces shame, shyness and embarrassment. Beyond the hegemonic discourse, which charged that children were too young to know about AIDS, Nicholas and Kayla suggested otherwise.

## Bullwood

| | |
|---|---|
| Nicholas: | I would wait for all the children to go and if we need to ask our teachers what is AIDS and they can tell you about it . . . And then you will know much more. Say that you are 8 years old and you have AIDS, you die at 16 but if you take medicine you live longer and longer. |
| DB: | Why would you wait for all the children to go? |
| Nicholas: | . . . Mrs Sing will tell us the full thing about AIDS. |
| DB: | . . . [B]ut why do you have to wait for everyone to be gone before you can ask Mrs Sing? |
| Nicholas: | . . . [Y]ou can by very, very shy. |
| Kayla: | I mean that there is parts of AIDS where it's really shy to talk about. |

AIDS invokes sexual shame, sexual stigma, embarrassment and shyness. Being embarrassed to talk about "parts of AIDS" functions as a means to discipline and regulate childhood innocence. The embarrassment that children feel about sex promotes and validates relations of power and children's place as innocent (Irvine 2002). However, children do have agency, and they do reflect on ways to manage the regulatory environment that curtails sexual knowledge. In this example, private discussions with the teacher it is suggested will alleviate the embarrassment and the shyness that many of the children spoke about when discussing AIDS and sex. Being shy and embarrassed to talk about the sexual parts of AIDS reproduces childhood innocence, but children can but exceed the boundaries through particular strategies they sought to adopt in their quest for knowledge.

Related to being embarrassed and shy was the focus on sexuality as funny and humorous. When children reflected on AIDS in the classroom, they interrogated a system of meaning in which sex was placed on the side of humour and laughter, suggesting that it was inappropriate for classroom discussions because children do not take it seriously:

| | |
|---|---|
| Dane: | I think that if you talk about sex stuff they're gonna go, errrrrrrrr [laughing loudly] . . . I don't know why. I think it's because they think that it's so stupid and it's funny and stuff like that. |

Laughter, humour, fun and giggles punctuated much of my discussions with children when it came to the sex part of AIDS and were constitutive of childhood sexualities (Allen 2014). Children are highly alert to the regulatory environment that diminishes their right to sexual knowledge. Laughter and humour function as an important technique for the regulation of childhood innocence. Children should feel shy about adult matters, but at the same time, laughter and humour break down sexuality as separate from childhood because it suggests children's active participation in sexual cultures that are derived from pleasure and excitement (Tobin 1997).

At Bullwood, the girls noted that the boys were particularly prone to react negatively to sex in AIDS education:

| | |
|---|---|
| DB: | Now tell me why only in high school? |
| Rita: | That's when they teach you a lot of things and that's when you understand and that's when you are bigger. |
| DB: | Don't you understand anything now? |
| Rita: | Just a little bit. |
| DB: | So the teacher should not talk to you about AIDS? |
| Rita: | No because some people are very rude and they always say horrible things and they say dirty things. |
| DB: | Like what tell me. Give me examples of dirty things. |
| Anne: | Like swearing and they say very horrible things. |
| DB: | Like who? |
| Rita: | I don't know. Maybe the boys. |
| DB: | What do they say? |
| Anne: | The 'B' word. |
| DB: | Who do they say it to? |
| Anne: | The girls . . . and they whisper into the each other's ears but they say it loud. They might say like something a swear word and say a knock-knock joke . . . and they might say a swear word. |

Measor, Tiffin and Fry (1996) suggest that it is boys in particular who use humour in sex education classes not only to suggest their displeasure but also to assert their masculine status. In the above example, the girls refer to the ways in which AIDS and teaching about sex could reproduce masculine power and authority through the use of "rude" words and the denigration of women and girls. AIDS education breaks a silence about sex, but discussion of sex could produce an environment where boys' reactions invoke relations of power based on gender/power imbalances and the repudiation of girls. In order to address this context, the girls suggest that AIDS education is more appropriate at a high school level because the humour and the sexual harassment would be disruptive. Humour operates to break the silence about sexuality. It complexly positions childhood sexuality on the side of shame and embarrassment, but it also suggests that sexuality is ever present, enjoyed and enjoyable. Enmeshed in the 'funny side' of sexuality, however, are oppressive gendered dynamics, and boys were particularly targeted for using jokes that were based on gsexual harassment and girls' subordination.

## Heterosexuality: Kissing and Boyfriends and Girlfriends

Heterosexual kissing and the association with boyfriends and girlfriends was also a complex source of pleasure and shame as it functioned to police and to explode notions of an acceptable childhood. As discussed in Chapter 2, popular notions of contagion permeated discussion around heterosexual kissing:

DB:      How do you get AIDS
Sophie:  Kissing . . . [Laughs]
DB:      How do you know that?
Sophie:  The disease goes into your mouth and that's how people have it.
Louis:   I heard something. I heard someone has AIDS. *Ja*, has AIDS . . . and he kissed that person on the lips and then she got AIDS!
Alice:   I don't really go near kissing faces. I wouldn't do it at all.
DB:      Why?
Alice:   It's because this school is a very good school. Right now you're not allowed to talk about girlfriends and boyfriends. Only in senior primary, you are allowed to.
Sophie:  I think high school.
Alice:   No, senior primary. And all the teachers say that you are not allowed to talk about boyfriends and girlfriends.
Sophie:  But I know some of the boys and girls—they have boyfriends and girlfriends.
Louis:   *Ja*, but they don't mention it, *ja*, it's like a boy has a friend, just a friend.

By asserting kissing as the transmission route of AIDS, the children re-assert into popular discourses of contagion and disease. Louis cites the example of someone he knows who kissed a "person on the lips and then she got AIDS!" Kissing (and its causal relationship with HIV risk) is dispelled to the domain of danger, shame and vulnerability. However, there is much more to this shaming. As seven- and eight-year-olds, the knowledge of sexual activity (and kissing) is considered inappropriate. The strategy to deal with this 'coming out' is to reject sexuality and to insert it within the discourse of shame. Recent work has established the ambivalence that young children demonstrate in the performance of sexuality distancing as an age-appropriate endeavour, giving meaning to innocence but also investing in sexuality by establishing heterosexual desirability and idealising heterosexual romance, boyfriends and girlfriends (Blaise 2005, 2010; Renold 2005). Children are thus active makers of sexuality whilst resisting and locking into discourses of innocence.

In the earlier transcripts, there is overt repulsion for the act of heterosexual kissing. Alice says, "I wouldn't do it at all". This is a justifiable response, particularly considering the risks involved in projecting an overt sexuality at the age of eight. As suggested, however, the ambiguity and contradictions of meaning around sexuality and the shame through which it is constructed are apparent. Dispelling kissing and constructing it in negative ways (its association with AIDS) is a strategic ploy to banish sexuality from their lives, project innocence and sustain popular accounts of the disease. Bullwood Primary School is constructed as a 'very good school' where sexual innocence is constructed as a marker of being 'good'. And yet, within the same discourse that attempts to position innocence, there are active heterosexual performances and contestation about when it is deemed appropriate to talk about heterosexual romance. Alice suggests senior primary whilst Sophie suggests "high school". Discussions about age-specific determinants around heterosexual romance function to police the boundaries of age and innocence. As the boys and girls give meaning to sex in AIDS, stigma operates in very complex ways as they stigmatise sex and sexuality as they police the acceptable boundaries of children's right to know sexually. The policing and shaming of sexuality is precisely the window to sexuality and the conversation illustrates the fragility of sexual innocence. Sophie and Louis confirm the existence of boyfriends and girlfriends breaking down the legitimacy of the 'good school'. It is also important to recognise that Louis suggested that boys and girls were friends, "just a friend". Consistent with other work on young children and sexuality in the primary school, the association of younger boys with girls can be constructed as contaminating and polluting, giving rise to homophobia (Renold 2005). Whilst older males invest in the production of a heterosexual masculinity and where the association with girls is desirable and a powerful assertion of masculinity, for younger boys at a stage where innocence is powerful, the association with girls as 'girlfriend' could be risky and have a stigmatising (homophobic) effect.

## KwaDabeka

Philani:   Sometimes they [girls] say silly thing like they say we look like cockroaches . . .

Sandile:   They call us flying cockroaches.

Lindo:   We also tease them . . . We say, "Hey you, mouse, go away from here" . . . [laughter]

At KwaDabeka, gendered dynamics operated through teasing and through which distance from boys and girls was constructed. Both boys and girls engaged in teasing each other, having fun in doing so but also subordinating each other. Whilst I did not witness physical fighting, boys stated that when girls teased them, they 'hit' back. AIDS education is thus produced in a context in which the effects are not transparent but complexly connected to a web of relations including age, gender, sex and contagion and involves policing and surveillance.

**WE SHOULD LEARN ABOUT AIDS**

Some children were of the opinion that they should learn about AIDS for their health and well-being:

## KwaDabeka

When young children talked about the need to talk about AIDS in the classroom the gendered nature of risk in a context of violence and poverty was clear:

> DB:       Should we talk about AIDS in the classroom?
> Pumzile:  We must talk about these things because sometimes you find that the child is being called by strangers and gets raped, so they will know that they must avoid strangers.

The vulnerability of young girls to rape is heightened in a context in which HIV is believed to be cured by having sex with a virgin (Leclerc-Madlala 2001). Here, Pumzile talks of powerlessness in relation to older men, which increases girls' risk of infection. Chapter 6 elucidates this further. Risk of HIV infection is compounded by the inability to negotiate safe sex and the centrality of gender and power in high risk associated with women (Bhana 2014). Pumzile's comments thus reflect a particular social reality, which makes urgent the need and the right to AIDS education. Children, Pumzile argues, must be told to avoid strangers because of the danger associated with strange men. The discourse of danger is thus heightened by affective imagery. While the danger facing young girls is clear in South Africa (Human Rights Watch 2001), the affective imagery works to reinforce innocence.

At Bullwood, the conversation highlighted the independence of young children by drawing on the potent symbol of blood, sickness, death and fear legitimising the need for AIDS education:

> Anton:    I think that we should learn about AIDS 'cause maybe when we grow up and we haven't learnt anything about AIDS then you don't know what it feels like to have AIDS and then you get it . . . and then you go to your doctor and you say feeling really unhappy. And then he asks that person a whole bunch of questions and then he answers yes to all of them and then he says well that's how it feels to have AIDS and you've got AIDS . . .
> DB:       Do you think we should talk to children about AIDS?
> Chorus:   Yes [together].
> DB:       Why?
> Damian:   It will make us more aware of AIDS. If you accidentally touch someone's blood then you know there is such a thing

|           | as AIDS, you can get AIDS but if you know what AIDS is you can be more careful. [Laughter] |
| --------- | --- |
| DB:       | Why should we know about AIDS? |
| Cassandra: | You'll know what AIDS is and you'd know how to get AIDS. You will be more careful. |
| Natalie:  | Because if don't know about it then if you could like get AIDS you don't know what's wrong with you you'll think it's a different kind of sickness and you think you're going to die straight away. |

In the preceding transcript the children at Bullwood, reinforce their capacity to rationalise and think, disrupting earlier representations of innocence. Not only is the assertion of their right to AIDS and health education being made clear, but the children also do so through psychological mechanisms combining fear and death and disease. Damian links AIDS with blood. The conversation has a serious tone. Blood and disease are ominous combinations. But the conversation quickly slips to laughter when he says, "If you *know what AIDS is* you can be more careful" (emphasis added). Here is an indication that if people know that AIDS is a sexually transmitted disease, then they can be more careful.

## CONCLUSION

This chapter was inspired by questions I raised in the research: "Should we talk about the disease?" and "Should your teachers/parents talk to you about it?" It was also inspired by the struggles of children's negotiation of their sexuality. I was always struck by how quickly narratives of knowing moved to not knowing and then knowing—a constant battle to live up to adult expectations whilst policing and policing each other. Children are very skilful, negotiating, resisting and adjusting their right to knowledge of sex, AIDS. The conversations with other boys and girls provided them with opportunities to display or hide their sexuality through a range of contradictory, gendered, 'age-appropriate' discourses. What this suggests is that given the right circumstances, children are very thoughtful and actively negotiate their own sexual predicaments, their pleasures and their concerns. Even at ages seven and eight, boys and girls are capable of reflecting on their actual lives and are happy to talk about AIDS and sexuality, but they are also acutely aware of being governed and controlled by discourses of innocence. As Walkerdine (2004) suggests, recourse to notions of childhood innocence in pedagogic discourses has the effect of turning displays of sexuality into something that is hidden, forbidden and subverted. To act and talk sexually are breaches of order and are forms of trouble themselves, and young children know this and are remarkable agents in managing adult concerns and anxieties.

In all, the chapter reveals the mockery of childhood innocence and the strategies that children devise to put adults at ease whilst their particular vulnerabilities are left unattended. People who have the greatest authority (parents and teachers) are often the least willing to speak about these matters. Some teachers have become so accustomed to dominant ideals of childhood that the living cultural worlds of young children are often ignored. In order to begin counteracting the threat to young children, teachers with proper training might open up discussion in the classroom and enable a more supportive environment, moving away from the preservation of sexual innocence and broadening the scope of young children's knowledge of AIDS, their vulnerability and their sexual and health well-being.

## REFERENCES

Allen, L. (2014) 'Don't Forget, Thursday Is Test[icle] Time! The Use of Humour in Sexuality Education'. *Sex Education*, 14(4): 387–399.
Banas, J., Dunbar, N., Rodriguez, D. & Liu. S. (2011) 'A Review of Humor in Educational Settings: Four Decades of Research'. *Communication Education*, 60(1): 115–144.
Barnes, C. (2012) 'It's No Laughing Matter . . . Boys' Humour and the Performance of Defensive Masculinities in the Classroom'. *Journal of Gender Studies*, 21(3): 239–251.
Blaise, M. (2005) *Playing it Straight: Uncovering Gender Discourses in the Early Childhood Classroom*. London: Routledge.
Blaise M (2010) 'Kiss and Tell: Gendered Narratives and Childhood Sexuality'. *Australasian Journal of Early Childhood*, 3(1): 1–9.
Bhana, D. (2014) *Under Pressure: The Regulation of Sexualities in South African Secondary Schools*. Mathoko's Books: Braamfontein.
Department of Education. (1996). *South African Schools Act*. Department of Education, Pretoria, South Africa.
Foucault, M. (1978) *The Will to Knowledge: The History of Sexuality, Volume 1* (Trans. R. Hurley). Penguin: Harmondsworth.
Human Rights Watch. (2001) *Scared at School: Sexual Violence Against Girls in South African Schools*. New York: Human Rights Watch.
Irvine, J. M. (2002) *Talk About Sex: The Battles Over Sex Education in the United States*. Berkeley: University of California Press.
James, A., Jenks, C. & Prout, A. (1998). *Theorising Childhood*. Cambridge: Polity.
Kehily, M. (ed). (2004) *An Introduction to Childhood Studies*. Buckingham: Open University Press.
Leclerc-Madlala, S. (2001). 'Virginity Testing: Managing Sexuality in a Maturing HIV/AIDS Epidemic'. *Medical Anthropology Quarterly*, 15(4): 533–552.
MacNaughton, G. (2000) *Rethinking Gender in Early Childhood Education*. London: Paul Chapman Publishing.
Measor, L., Tiffin, C. & Fry, K. (1996) 'Gender and Sex Education: A Study of Adolescent Responses'. *Gender and Education*, 8(3): 275–288.
Renold, E. (2005) *Girls, Boys and Junior Sexualities*. London: Routledge Falmer.
Robinson, K. (2013) *Innocence, Knowledge and the Construction of Childhood: The Contradictory Nature of Sexuality and Censorship in Children's Contemporary Lives*. New York: Routledge.

Silin, J. (1995) *Sex, Death and the Education of Children: Our Passion for Ignorance in the Age of AIDS*. New York: Teachers College Press.

Thorne, B. (1993) *Gender Play: Girls and Boys in School*. New Brunswick, NJ: Rutgers University Press.

Tobin, J. (ed) (1997) *Making a Place for Pleasure in Early Childhood Education*. New Haven, CT: Yale University Press.

Walkerdine, V. (2004) 'Development Psychology and the Study of Childhood', in M. Kehily. (ed) *An Introduction to Childhood Studies* (pp. 96–107). Buckingham: Open University Press.

# 6  AIDS, not Sex! Teaching Innocence

Kirsty:  We would have to talk about AIDS if Mrs Hobbs said that 'cause we have to listen to our teachers.
DB:      And if says, you can't?
Kirsty:  Only if she says we can, then we can talk about it.
Emma:    . . . '[C]ause it's a serious thing and we have to talk about it.
DB:      And who should be talking to us about it?
Kirsty:  Our parents and our teachers.
Emma:    Our parents . . .

—Discussion with eight-year-olds Kirsty and Emma at Bullwood

Sex is at the heart of AIDS (Boyce *et al.* 2007). Sex is also at the heart of AIDS education producing the paradox between the desire to uphold the innocence of childhood and the critical importance of addressing what is at the heart of AIDS and sex. This chapter begins with conversations I had with children about who should talk to them about AIDS. Emma and Kirsty at Bullwood suggested that it was their teachers and parents. If children thought that adults had a role to play in AIDS education, how do they approach the children's AIDS-related knowledge? This chapter is concerned with the discussions I had with teachers at Bullwood and KwaDabeka. When I first embarked on this study, the chief focus was on young children's constructions of gender and sexuality in their AIDS-related knowledge. However, as I described in Chapter 1, I found myself talking to teachers and asking them questions about their role in facilitating sexual knowledge of the disease. They said children were "not yet ready". This reluctance forms the major focus of discussion in this chapter. The assumption in this study, like that of Epstein and Johnson (1998), is that it is ridiculous to assume that children do not draw conclusions from the visible and invisible sexuality of adults and children around them. In fact, along with Watney (1991) researchers should not be debating whether children are sexual beings, but we should be concerning ourselves with the ways in which adults respond to childhood sexuality. This chapter focuses on adult teachers' deployment of childhood innocence in constructing children's AIDS-related knowledge.

In Chapter 8 I focus on mothers' approach to and practices related to the of children's AIDS-related knowledge.

Throughout the world, the subject of childhood sexuality education commonly produces deep anxiety and is intensely contested (Robinson 2013). As I have argued in this book, childhood innocence remains a hegemonic adult discourse. According to this view, children should be protected from corrupting information related to the sexual world of adults; they should have little or preferably no sexual knowledge that could damage their innocence or tempt them into 'forbidden' practices (Renold 2005). The presumption of innocence means immunity from sexual knowledge and this imbues the adult with knowledge and power in the need for children to be protected from the supposedly pernicious influences of the adult sexual world.

In South Africa the seriousness of the AIDS pandemic and the efforts to contain and prevent its spread has opened up the possibility of dealing with sexuality in the primary school and including it within the life skills curriculum. There is a strong argument that teachers are very important in mediating children's knowledge about sexuality, sexual health and AIDS (Miedema *et al.* 2015). However, fundamental questions remain about how teachers construct children's right to knowledge about sex as part of AIDS education and how various discourses are deployed in dealing with its complexity. Recent research has suggested that practising teachers asked to teach about AIDS may experience considerable embarrassment and anxieties about sexuality (Namisi *et al.* 2009; Francis 2012; Iyer & Aggleton 2013; Wood & Rolleri 2014). Teachers may not be sure of what to teach, how to teach it and fail to address the right of children to open and honest sexual expression (Pattman & Chege 2003; Miedema *et al.* 2015). AIDS interventions in schools appear to be missing the message, ignoring boys' and girls' different responses to knowledge about AIDS and be blind to the construction of gendered and sexual identities (Morrell *et al.* 2009). In the context of childhood sexuality education, where sexuality is taboo, teachers may be drawing on familiar and taken-for-granted assumptions about the role of a teacher in AIDS-related knowledge (Silin 1995). Underlying this uneasiness are longstanding conventions that associate children with innocence. The image of the naturally asexual, pure child is at the heart of teachers' reluctance to engage with the topic of sex as part of AIDS education. As the previous chapter has shown, the persistent conceptualisation of children as sexually innocent makes it difficult for children to assert sexual agency or for adults to accept the existence of sexuality in children. Adult power is often institutionalised in schools, leaving children with little opportunity in official encounters to bring up the topic of sex. Mellor and Epstein (2006) report that while children do resist discussions, adults are often in charge, producing a discursive context where 'adults are teachers' and 'children are learners'. This relationship has numerous implications for AIDS education. Teachers are strategically positioned to mediate learners' knowledge about sex; they are also powerful agents producing and reproducing what is taught in AIDS education and how it is taught in the classroom (Baxen & Breidlid 2009).

Teaching discourses involve contradictory ways of relating to young children's right to knowledge about AIDS in their upholding of the notion of the innocent child and in their reproduction of gender inequalities. Teachers' responses also tap into what Kincaid (1994) calls "hard-core righteous prurience" about sexuality and children. Childhood sexuality functions to produces shame, contempt and disgust by teachers (and adults), and this is a strategic advantage held by teachers to prevent the possibility of linking AIDS to sex and sexuality and constraining efforts to teach more comprehensively about AIDS and prevention in the primary curriculum. Instead of being able to respond to, and participate in, AIDS-prevention programmes, sex and sexuality are excluded based on adult monopolistic narratives of childhood innocence. Heinze (2000) suggests that adults often draw upon the discourse of childhood innocence to uphold particular images of childhood, producing and protecting the ideal child as innocent, asexual and degendered.

Children are assumed to be immune to (if not victims of) sexual knowledge and representation. Appeals to protect innocent children, especially their sexual innocence, wield a great deal of power (Irvine 2002). AIDS education triggers feelings of fear and disgust amongst teachers and the emotions are deployed ambivalently to reproduce the innocent child. Teachers draw contradictorily on affective conventions of fear and anxiety in which sex is taboo and sexuality too dangerous to be countenanced in childhood (Tobin 1997). The contradiction is the desire to uphold sexual innocence but also recognition that young children are sexual agents; otherwise, why bother about the fear of sexuality? It must be noted, too, that teachers can be easily stigmatized by their perceived associations with sex, should they be known to talk about sex, and such associations in relation to young children can be seen to be highly suspect by parents and the wider community.

The teachers in this chapter, like the boys and girls in this study, emerge from vastly different social contexts where race and class has had effects for the presence of AIDS and who suffers from the adverse outcomes of the disease. How the innocence of children is constructed is not random or spontaneous but manifests the social and political context through which childhood is experienced. Thus, the relationship of many teachers to the subject of childhood sexuality and AIDS education is inscribed within regulatory forces based on the notion of childhood innocence which uphold and construct a version of childhood but which is racialised, classed and gendered. Despite the urgency of addressing young children as active agents and with knowledge of AIDS and sex, the discourse of childhood innocence is mobilized by teachers in both primary schools and culminates in fear and anxiety around the expression of childhood sexuality.

In this chapter, interviews conducted with teachers illustrate the dominance of childhood innocence. Mrs Hobbs (white) and Mrs Sing (Indian) at Bullwood and Mrs Shange, Mrs Thusi and Ms Sishi (all African) at KwaDabeka are the teachers of the children in this study. This was followed by further interviews with Ms Burke (white) at Bullwood and Mr Xaba (African) at KwaDabeka about two years after the initial interviews when children were in grade 4—many of whom were in their classes. Throughout my conversation with Mr Xaba, he often referred to sex as "that word" refusing to say sex only repeating "that word", or through spelling it out: s–e–x. It is argued that childhood sexuality and AIDS education reveals a paradox. Despite the need to engage with knowledge and information about the disease, discourses of childhood innocence are bolstered working to deny, silence and repress the heart of AIDS and sex. Teaching discourses are conservative and hegemonic, and they work against children's agency and expression of sexuality. The chapter identifies several interlocking discursive strategies through which children's knowledge of the relationship between sex and AIDS is regulated through development theory but also through context specific narratives that are the effects of structural and social inequalities. While teachers' constructions of childhood innocence are formidable, they are not irreversible because teachers point in contradictory ways to young children's sexual agency. The significance of starting early with young children, together with the calamitous effects of AIDS in South Africa, indicates that researchers must begin confronting the AIDS pandemic and start to develop AIDS reduction and prevention programmes appropriate to the early years of schooling.

## BULLWOOD AND KWADABEKA: AIDS, NOT SEX

Silin (1995) argues that too much of the contemporary childhood curriculum brings a deadly silence to the being of childhood and not enough of it speaks to things that really matter to children's lives. AIDS matters in childhood and so does sex. When teachers in this study were asked about the importance of sex in AIDS education they constructed themselves in ambivalent ways. The ambivalence is evident in the ways respect to children is meant to by denying and/or limiting reference to sex but at the same time use the discourse of innocence to construct and perpetuate their authority and power over children.

## Bullwood

Primary school is often seen as a social and cultural site producing and signifying innocence (Walkerdine 2004). In the theory of development, for example, children are often constructed as adults 'in the making' (Thorne 1993) and thus still asexual. Innocence marks and separates young children from older childhoods (e.g. secondary school experience) and from adults. The context of AIDS education presents an ideal space through which to understand the adult/teacher gaze on the child. At Bullwood 'too young to know' was firmly established amongst the teachers as an argument for refusing to address sexuality related AIDS education:

> Sing:  I don't think that they know too much about HIV/AIDS. I think that it's just a few of them that know but generally 'cause you can't really talk about it. I mean, as their teacher, I would not want to get too much into that 'cause they're too small. Children should not be introduced to this sort of thing at such an early age. They're too young and then they start to experiment . . . that is why I would not like to sort of talk about sex . . . If they ask any question, I give them innocent answers . . . they don't really know about it or sex. They're very innocent. So we don't talk too much about it. We don't say much about it. They just know it's a disease . . . and I feel . . . I belong to the old-fashion[ed] school of thought. Children should not be introduced to this sort of thing at such an early age. They are too young and then they start to experiment . . . I would not like to sort of talk about sex . . . or anything relating to sex in class. If they ask any question, I give them innocent answers.

According to the teacher, all children need to know (and what they do know is the disease AIDS) but beyond that their innocence is presented as paramount. There are contradictions, however. Sing admits that her views belong to an "old-fashion[ed] school of thought". It is not that children do not know sex; otherwise, why would she be concerned about the expression of sexual agency through experimentation? Whilst there has been objection to the notion that sexual talk leads to sexual experimentation (Stone *et al.* 2013), the point here is that Sing does not like to talk about sex-related issues in AIDS education.

This is confirmed by Burke:

> I didn't want to get into that aspect [sex]; and maybe at a higher level, as they get older, that could be touched on; because they are very innocent at this age and I just feel that it's just too, too much for them; and they get, they get silly and they can't, I don't know, they can't handle the conversation, if you know what I mean . . . I taught sexuality education in the UK for a long, fair amount of time, and I just feel that at this age they are far too young; they really are so.

Burke presents herself as experienced in the issues of sexuality education as she mentions she had taught it, not only in South Africa but also in the

United Kingdom, for a "fair amount of time". She positions herself not only as knowledgeable in the area of sexuality and childhood, but she also confirms and contributes to the discourse of sexual innocence by claiming that children cannot manage conversations around the topic of sex. The idea that children are too young to know about sexuality implies that older children do know. Burke's argument about the "higher level" makes pedagogical sense to her, and it can be associated with a developmental approach that has widespread approval in teacher training (see MacNaughton 2000). A developmental approach, as suggested earlier, is based on incremental and linear unfolding and development of identity within social contexts. Adults have power, and children are assumed to not know about sexuality, but it is also assumed that they ought not to know.

Childhood sexuality is created in relation to adult sexuality, and the two are imbued with power relations and are in opposition to each other. When the teachers in this study were asked why they were reluctant to engage with the topic of sex in AIDS education, they drew on sex displacing strategies. For example, Burke remarked,

> As I've said, I've taught sexuality education for the past five years in the UK, so I'm quite happy with it, but it's a completely different world here . . . But I do feel that they are very young, and especially back in South Africa, if I compare the level of the kids to [those in] the UK, I feel the UK [children] are far more, they are older and they're, they're more, I don't know, possibly more mature, and more they're faced with a lot more issues; whereas these kids I feel are a little more protected, and that's why I think they need a little bit of time, you know, and because it's a sort of an introduction to the whole HIV thing. I think that possibly even next year or the year after . . . I think that would be a more perfect time to discuss with them about the sexual aspect of HIV.

AIDS education draws together complex social meanings around sexuality including ones involving race and space. The South African landscape is a peculiar example of not only how the "racial becomes the spatial" (Pred 2000: 98) but also how race/space/class and AIDS are intimately connected. Burke invests in a version of an idealised South African landscape, which she viewed as a "completely different world"; sexuality education in the UK was considered more appropriate, because children there had to deal with "more issues". The global culture in the United Kingdom has possibly created moral panic about the 'disappearance of childhood' and notions of the sexually corrupt child (Renold 2005). These moments of moral panic hinge primarily on the issue of early sexual maturation, which is viewed as a particular threat to childhood. Within the context of the global UK culture, Burke perceived a hurried sexuality among schoolchildren; in that context she saw sexuality education as appropriate and necessary for dealing with overly sexualized young children. And, she contrasted the sexual freedom in the United Kingdom and the hurried sexuality of children there with a particular understanding of South African childhood and its social reality. The South African social reality is that HIV prevalence has resulted in devastating effects, increasing children's vulnerabilities as a result of AIDS deaths and increasing morbidity and heightening the demands made on children to care for family members infected or affected by HIV.

However, it is important to understand the variegated experiences of South African children. By drawing on race/space/class and the various understandings of childhood located in these constructs, Burke was able to legitimise sexual silence, for predominantly white South African schoolchildren. Her statements suggest that she perceives AIDS as a disease of the 'other,' mostly African and poor, and as something located in spaces constructed by apartheid and still separating rich from poor and white from African. Thus, Burke constructs innocence, framing it by an idealisation of middle-class white South African childhood innocence and separating it from the decadence of the global sexual freedoms of childhood in the United Kingdom, as well as the spectre of the black South African township context of the disease. Unlike the children she taught at Bullwood Primary School, who presumably needed to be protected from frank discussions of sex and AIDS, she felt that the children she had taught in the United Kingdom apparently already possessed considerable sexual knowledge; this allowed Burke to feel satisfied that topical issues around sex cannot matter to young white children in the middle class and, by implication, that their context helped guarantee their safety from HIV infection.

## At KwaDabeka

Mr Xaba acknowledges a specific context at KwaDabeka that highlights the need for sexuality education:

> [A]t the workshop they stressed that we should call a spade a spade, because there was a case in a court whereby a pupil wanted to lay a rape charge on her uncle. She kept referring to the penis as a carrot, so at the time they laid a charge at the police station the statement read—he showed me his carrot so the man was acquitted. The girl was afraid to say penis and so she kept saying carrot.

While there is a general recognition of the value of sexuality education, the prevailing discourses of sexuality and sexual language still incite fear and shame. Irvine (2002) shows how initiatives to regulate sexual speech in education can be fuelled by the idea that sexual language can trigger social chaos and result in anarchy. Irvine adds that words denoting sexuality produce anxiety in adults because they are tainted by their association with actual sexual practices. On the whole, the regulation of sexual speech produces sex as a domain of danger and shame. Despite official departmental training where Xaba learned to call 'a spade, a spade', sex is not sex but is displaced. When asked when it was appropriate to say *sex* to children, Xaba responded,

> Maybe at the age of 16 or 17. The children become very active because of the diet, these dairy products like cheese they eat, and they develop breasts, then so we should teach them at that age. So 16 to 18 is okay.

Despite recognising the discussion of sexuality as an integral part of AIDS education teacher training and classroom lessons, Xaba displaced the topic of sex to a relation to age and biology (gender). Workshops on teaching AIDS education, such as the one he attended, can create a context where teachers like Xaba are expected to disrupt normative assumptions about sexuality in childhood.

However, discourses of biology linked to developmental discourses are widely influential in the ways in which teachers tie themselves to (and are themselves tied to) the idea of childhood as a time of sexually immature phenomena.

Xaba suggests that the attainment of sexual maturity, between the ages of 16 and 18, warrants education related to sexual activity but not sooner. This strategy is related to dominant discourses that tend to construct children as biologically and sexually immature and without the knowledge or the capacity to think, act or understand sexually. Children who deviate from this notion of sexual and biological innocence are pathologised. In Xaba's view, children's diet (dairy products) can increase sexual maturation and hence sexual activity, while that pathologisation is also highly gendered, making girls' sexuality visible (breasts) but not that of boys. It is often argued that boys are rarely subject to the hurried-child discourse, while girls are—through comments like "She's a woman before her time" (Janssen 2002; Renold 2005). Xaba's comments on diet, breasts and sexual activity likewise contribute to this.

At KwaDabeka, AIDS, but not sex, was permeated by notions of respect but was underpinned by discursive strategies to uphold childhood innocence:

> Thusi: The culture is respect, respect. If you respect children you can't talk to children about sex. I'm not deep about sex. We can talk about AIDS, not sex. I say you can get infected and you mustn't sleep with somebody but no further detail.

The distinct marker between adult teacher and child is respect and this is achieved and guaranteed by making sex off limits. Sexual silence signals respect. The focus on AIDS, not sex, reflects the recourse to the notion of childhood innocence. This recourse does not happen in automatic ways. Thusi says, "You mustn't sleep with somebody", thus hinting at sex, but she cannot or will not say the word *sex*. By invoking respect for children she identifies herself and orientates herself in particular ways in relation to children which privilege her role as their protector against dangerous sexual knowledge:

> Sishi:   No I won't be comfortable to talk about sex; I will be comfortable to talk about AIDS. I'll speak freely without boundaries without recognizing their age I will talk freely. This disease is around and there is nothing to hide but when you speak about sex . . . *ai*, it will give me trouble. Once I spoke about sex, I never get straight. I gave them fear. I said that "if you do this, you're going to get AIDS. You're going to get infected with AIDS. Have you seen people with AIDS?" They've got diarrhoea, maggots to make them fear. That's why I say I cannot teach sex because I know what I'm going to say to them.

Talk about AIDS and sex provokes silence, denial and shame. Sex in the context of AIDS is being produced as a negative domain of danger and fear. Sishi reinforces the AIDS-not-sex discourse—by disassociating HIV from sex she articulates her own anxieties ("trouble") in relation to sex and young children. When she spoke of AIDS, on the other hand, she constructed herself as free and as without fear and anxiety: "This disease is around and there is nothing to hide".

Research on secondary teachers and AIDS education points out that the biomedical model—or the information-based approach—is based on teachers presenting facts (Campbell 2003). This factual approach has been seen to be unsuccessful because children's lives and realities are of peripheral concern. In contrast to the information-based approach, Sishi resorts to imparting misinformation, thus inducing fear and disgust by using inflammatory images (maggots) to evoke powerlessness amongst young children, and she thus conceals sexuality behind fear and danger. Sishi invokes images of evil, contamination and dirt, which are perceived as indicators of the diseased AIDS body (diarrhoea and maggots). Sishi's comments thus work to secure a distancing from the disease through psychologically manipulative mechanisms, including fear. Sex is constructed as dangerous, something to be feared, taboo and forbidden, and punishable by disease: "if you do this, you're going to get AIDS". The result of sex is AIDS, diarrhoea, maggots and death. This fosters ominous fantasies, and these fantasies are indicators of both individual and social vulnerability. There is the wilful dissemination of misinformation about the disease in order to maintain distance from the guilty and thus protect the innocent child from corruption (Mayall 2002). The result is thus not only to control or eliminate sexual discussion but also to construct sex as evil/bad and that which necessarily produces AIDS. Sishi cannot talk about sex as pleasure because this equation cannot be reconciled with the rhetoric and promotion of childhood innocence. She speaks of sex but in terms of terrible consequences. Childhood sexuality is thus regulated and policed through a system of opposition: sex is constructed as danger/germs/death and innocence as purity and freedom from these horrors. Yet there are implicit assumptions here that children are indeed sexual beings, otherwise why bother with AIDS education that is framed around warnings about the dangers of having sex? And, of course, Sishi is clear when she talks about young children having sex; however, she constructs these children as the 'naughty' ones, thus making it clear that the children do know about sex. The construction of the naughty/innocent opposition serves to uphold innocence as normal and naughtiness (with sexual knowledge) as pathological. This is discussed in the next part of this section.

Similarly, Xaba's understanding of AIDS education was premised upon the notion of innocence, culture respect and cultural constructs:

> I keep on avoiding some of the things that I said, like in our custom, there are something we are tabooed, like that word I mentioned, like s–e–x . . . I think, because in our custom, we as blacks, it's still very difficult to mention the word sex, especially to a person of young age, especially we as the torchbearers; they will think that we are encouraging them to do this thing, to be sexually active. We grew up in these families where this is taboo, and we have to follow whatever we are told. Our tradition goes a very long way, because, right now, I'm still afraid of talking and telling my smaller brother about that word, although I can see that he is sexually active. The only thing I do is to make them aware that the disease is here, and either you are infected or affected, and maybe we can see neighbours' family have AIDS, and let them know of dos and don'ts. The pupils here, it's their age and their level, and they may misinterpret what I'm saying, and they may think that he is encouraging us, and they might say that they want to experience this thing, because Mr Xaba mentioned this thing, and it's OK to do this thing, but at their age they should abstain.

This construction fuses cultural anxieties about sexuality with panic about childhood sexuality, and in doing so demonstrates the complicated mechanisms of regulation in childhood sexuality. Culture and race may be appropriated and reworked to split off and marginalise the topic of sex from AIDS education. Invoking culture and race in deterministic ways produces a static logic concerning childhood sexuality, which prevents teachers (like Xaba) from engaging in issues related to sexuality. Generational hierarchies embedded within the practices of *ukuhlonipha* are important in making sense of the culturally acceptable behaviour that precludes discussion of sex and reasserts age categories and relations. Zulu cultural practices called *ukuhlonipha* can also be linked to the avoidance of conversations with young children about sex. Hunter (2010) refers to *ukuhlonipha* as customs of avoidance and deference, which reflect generational divisions, but these are also contested and reinforced. Talking about sex to children challenges *ukuhlonipha*, and so it is more comfortable for a teacher to resist engagement with the topic of sex nor sexuality and thus feed into *ukuhlonipha*. Xaba added,

[I]f they bring it [sex] up I will answer it, but I don't want to get in-depth, because kids are fairly innocent. I was beating around the bush in the classroom when I asked them how AIDS [*sic*] is spread. I wanted them to tell me, but maybe I think they are afraid because the word sex, kissing, touching private parts, all those things, they are not allowed to mention those words, though it's happening.

"It's happening" offers the room to reconsider development approaches. Even static conceptions of race and culture, like developmental discourses, are not as fixed, as Xaba suggested, but are open to alternate possibilities. In fact, childhood reality, as Xaba stated, goes against such fixed conceptions of the child. Fear and anxiety are important psychological tools invested in the sexual regulation of childhood. The fear of parents, for example, is key to policing the boundaries of children's sexual innocence. Xaba's anxieties about sexuality in childhood stem from the relationship between sexual information and sexual stimulation. The horror of imagining sexuality education with sex stimulation is heightened within the context of a township primary school. Sears (1992) describes how teachers resort to teaching sex as a series of facts, driven by the fear of attack induced by saying the word *sex*.

In a South African context, where the behaviour of some male teachers in townships has contributed to the relatively high level of sexual violence against girls, Xaba's fears are not groundless (see Human Rights Watch 2001). Teachers, and males in particular, who mention sex in such contexts can be more or less 'presumed guilty until proven innocent.' Xaba's fear as a teacher may derive from a sense of his vulnerability in the school and in the community, where male teachers are under increasing scrutiny for sexual abuse. The mechanisms of sexual regulation have many components, both in and outside of education. Xaba mentions his relationship with his younger brother, and so drawing on *ukuhlonipha*. The inability to say *sex* derives from deep-rooted traditions, which are seen as impermeable.

The effect is the pronouncement only of basic instructions, 'dos and don'ts,' which work to preserve sexual innocence, while misrecognising children's sexual agency and reinvesting in age hierarchies, culture and race to construct the adult as 'torchbearers.' Specific cultural practices create the conditions for what is possible in teaching young children and have severe impacts on the information made available to them. For Xaba, this also had an impact on how he dealt with his younger brother.

## KWADABEKA: NAUGHTY/INNOCENT CHILDREN

AIDS is embedded within a system of representation that is constituted by ideologically defined dichotomies such as good/bad. Fuss (1989: 103) says this best in her observation that "identity is always purchased at the price of the exclusion of the Other". At KwaDabeka, the naughty/innocent dichotomy is illustrative of the exclusion of the other-naughty who has sexual knowledge:

> There are naughty ones in the class. They talked about sex play. Sex is 'hide and seek'. They play 'hide and seek'. They say, "*Blekimapatile*, where are you?" This play is play sex. When they play there are some naughty ones then they will do sex . . . six-, seven- even five-year olds, even in this school. There was another teacher here and she had a child in the preschool then she said, "Mummy, I saw somebody doing sex at school". They see this from their parents. My daughter I never wanted her to mix. When she was young I knew there is something bad you cannot take away from the kids so I sent her to Thomas More [a private school in Durban]. I knew that kids experience this game. I knew that children reported sex to me. (Sishi)

Sexual innocence is not the domain of young children, but it is wished on them by teachers. The preceding extract clearly indicates that childhood innocence is a myth: children play at sex and have even reported sexual activity to Sishi.

Advocating AIDS education but not sexuality education was an important means through which teachers identified and defined themselves and through which a version (or illusion) of the innocent child was sustained. Yet sex play and sexual activity in the school enter the teachers' conversation, and this triggers tension and anxiety about the fact of children's sexual curiosity. Children's sexual agency, while recognised (and repressed), is regulated under the category 'naughty' while other children (and her own child, too) are constructed as innocent. Sishi decries naughty children—those with sexual knowledge—but sees this as endemic to the township school. Not only does the dichotomy work to position innocent and naughty children, but it works, too, to position good and bad schools and good and evil childhoods. Her knowledge of sexual activity amongst young children and her desire to distance herself from this meant that she uprooted her child from the township school to send her to Thomas More—a private, elite and predominantly white school in Durban. Sexuality becomes a negative domain of danger and immorality in the township school regulated through race and class constructs. Her daughter becomes the representation of the very state of purity from which she must never be removed and which must be protected so she is sent to a private predominantly white school. Working-class African children with sexual knowledge are seen to be threats to childhood innocence. KwaDabeka Primary School and Thomas More become disreputable and respectable respectively, and naughty children are constructed as unhealthy and infectious. This reinforces the regulatory system controlling childhood through the mechanism of the notion of innocence. Implicit in this conversation is disgust and contempt for the naughty child.

These affective conventions of sexuality, which guide thinking about young children, reinforce sexual shame and attempt to preserve innocence.

By invoking moralistic injunctions, Sishi has presented her innocent child in contrast to those who engage in sex play and sexual activities. Not only are these other children the bad versions of childhood, but she is also someone who is morally and socially superior to the naughty children in her classroom. By extension Sishi presents herself, as the child's parent, as occupying a similar position:

> Sishi:    It's because they are young. Even their parents don't talk about sex. Young, very young. They should be told but the parents should help, because some parents say that sex should not be taught to our kids. They never got contact with different kids. I have now 16 years of experience. I know kids. No one can tell me about kids. If you talk about sex you have to be aware of their age. I've heard from our department that there should be levels of development but our kids even nine years know something above your age. If you're 25 years old, they know more than you but now the department restricts you but now it cannot work in that way. They already know. Parents don't care. Kids are neglected by their parents. Some of the kids enjoy sex. There was a little girl in my class now she's in grade 5. She has been involved since grade 1. Can you imagine? I heard the story from other kids and from the granny. This one was abused by the uncle and this uncle was sent to jail and then I said to her, "Why didn't you tell me?" and she said, "I was afraid, I was afraid".

Defending sexuality education and talk about the subject in early schooling can be extremely dangerous especially in the context where parents and the department of education do not provide support for AIDS education in schools and sexuality education. Sishi makes clear the regulatory forces both from the department that guides teacher's work and from the parents. Significantly, there are strong resonances in this conversation of theories that relate early sexual experience to cultural deprivation.

Children who engage in sex are seen as coming from bad homes with bad parents who do not care and who are irresponsible. "Some of the children enjoy sex" is articulated against assumed sexual innocence by drawing on an emotional performance associated with disgust and contempt in relation to naughty children. Sishi's comment on children who enjoy sex serves to stigmatize and exclude them because of their nonconformity to the ideal. Sexually precocious children are seen to be naughty and this is problematic. Recognizing that children "already know" is a powerful contradiction, in some ways, to the force of assumed innocence. Childhood sexuality is thus being thought about in conflicting and contradictory ways: children do not know, and they already know. These contradictions occur within the set of emotional responses that guide conventions about appropriate forms of childhood. For example, childhood sex is linked in Sishi's mind to the abuse of children and to bad parenting. Her recounting the response: "I was afraid, I was afraid" is a powerful emotional response to the innocence of young children—girls in particular—and their need for protection, and it works, too, to induce panic about children's sexuality. Very often in South Africa, the only discussion of children and sexuality takes place in the context of child abuse. Because of the high rates of child sexual abuse there is certainly a need to address this issue in South Africa (Richter *et al.* 2004), but this must be done without demonizing childhood sexuality (as this teacher is doing) and associating it necessarily with abuse. Sishi laments the grade 5 child's loss of innocence in her trying to uphold the romanticised version of sexual innocence. Actually it is precisely because childhood sexuality is so taboo a subject that children are particularly vulnerable to child sexual abuse.

## KWADABEKA: POLARISING BOYS AND GIRLS IN AIDS EDUCATION

Childhood innocence is deeply gendered with girls' innocence being eroticized (Walkerdine 2004). In South Africa, young virgin girls have been raped due to the myth that having sex with a virgin will cure the AIDS disease. The eroticisation of little girls provokes adult concern for their protection and the price of their innocence is too high. The teachers at KwaDabeka in the study placed a great deal of significance on gender, with girls' vulnerability being an important concern in AIDS education:

Thusi:   Sometimes they get raped. They have to run away from adults because they can rape them, especially the girls. They can get AIDS and we have to tell them about AIDS. I tell them that AIDS is a disease that you get from having sex with others.

In her statement, young girls are made vulnerable, are victimized and are constructed as defenceless. Adult men are homogenized and described as predatory. Masculine sexuality becomes emblematic of male power and is expressed through sexual violation. While rape is part of the harsh reality of present-day South Africa, where many girls continue to be vulnerable, the effect of seeing girls as quintessentially defenceless victims is to construe them necessarily as existing without power or agency. Moreover, knowledge about sex and AIDS is premised on the dangerous force of sexuality. Young girls are thus homogenized as being the innocent victims of adult men who have AIDS rather than as active participants in their gender and sexual identity.

The emotional template in this instance operates to produce the poor girl victim. Threatened rape and imagined dangers to girls produce a climate in which anxiety and fear are produced. This is not to deny that girls are raped and that women and girls are victims of sexual violence, but her comments reinforce only the sexual vulnerability of girls, and they assume that girls who do go around with boys are bad girls. Her comments construe boy/girl relationships as inevitably sexual, and they deny the possibility of boys and girls mixing as friends.

When asked if boys and girls can work together in AIDS education the teachers focused on gender differences and the polarisation of gender identities:

> Shange:   The boys know that I'm a boy and the girls know that. Even if you mix them they want to be boys only and girls only I just say that you have to mix just to kill that stereotype. If they are outside in the break they separate. You get the rare case of the boy playing with the girl. Girlish boys. There is a boy in my class who is girlish. He is friend to girls. The other boys say, "You are this, you are this—'*isitabane*' [sissy]". There are four boys who are bullies. They hit everybody, they take others' belongings, and they make fun of others. If someone teases them there is a fight.

Shange refers to the problems of boys. Shange shows how boys are the problem, and this is based on their less-than-satisfactory behaviour. Her own beliefs about sissies reinforce gender polarities. The polarised description of boys and girls works to constrain teachers in exercising power and in ensuring a more gender-harmonious classroom that benefits all. Shange's focus on bad boys serves to legitimate masculine power, thus disempowering her as far as changing gender relations in the classroom in concerned: the possibility for dialogue and friendships across the genders is erased and, with it, the possibility of change. While Shange refers to varied forms of masculinity in her classroom, for example the *isitabane*, boys are lumped together as violent beings and this serves to reproduce unequal gender power relations:

> Thusi:   Our culture, I don't know how if I love you as a boy I'll always ill treat you, I don't know. I always see boys ill treat girls that they love, he grabs her, and he kicks her, I don't know why. If he loves you he will ill treat you. The young ones they know that. Boys know that.

The effects of these constructions of boys and girls are deeply problematic because the implication is that boys are monsters and that girls should keep away from them. Heterosexual love is dangerous and it has violent effects. While there are certainly high rates of gender violence in South Africa, there is also the pathological positioning of girls as victims and a sense of resignation that boys (even young boys), who know their power and status in heterosexual relations, are necessarily violent. Within the particular context of KwaDabeka the specific discourses on 'culture' and particular practices are appropriated and reworked, thus having an impact on the nature of social relations in the classroom. A central issue here is that Thusi inscribes boys with power by engaging with cultural forms that validate asymmetrical heterosexual relations of power. Here it is assumed that neither boys nor girls have the power to change their positions in society because of cultural discourses and practices. Girls and women are rendered as passive, unprotesting victims of culture and thus as power-less victims. In this way particular positions are inhabited based on the cultural practices that marginalise others and are particularly damaging to girls.

## BULLWOOD AND KWADABEKA: ANXIETIES ABOUT PARENTS

> Hobbs: It's quite a tricky one. I don't do anything except health is-sues. It's a tricky one. I believe that parents are not comfort-able with us doing their job. Actually I don't think that the kids know one person who has it. Also at the senior primary level there's lots of experts that talk about explicit stuff but I think they're too young to be told issues. I do say, "Don't touch others, don't take suckers from others" but these are basic hygiene stuff. But no, I belong to a mothers' group and, no, parents will not be comfortable with this.

Defending topics relating to sexual activity in the context of AIDS educa-tion can be precarious, especially in the context where not only the icon of the asexual child is pervasive but also where parental oversight of teachers' work in schools is increasing. In South Africa, for example, parental power has increased in many decisions that schools make about teacher appoint-ments and school policies, even to the extent of determining uniform policy (Department of Education 2005). Mr Xaba shows how the association with classroom discussions about sex can produce fear as a result of parental hostility:

> Yes, I'm very afraid to mention those words because sometimes they will tell their parents that so and so was teaching us about s–e–x, and they will storm me with phone calls, and maybe some of the parents will come to the school and accuse me of giving bad information to the pupils.

The anarchy that could result from parental dissent around 'bad infor-mation' is an important factor regulating AIDS education in the primary school classroom. Speaking about sex is viewed negatively by parents, and in the specific context of KwaDabeka, it seems it could have provoked major confrontation with teachers. Teachers' fear and anxiety induced by parental objection function to regulate and limit what information can and cannot be stated in HIV/AIDS education lessons. Childhood sexuality thus produces and is invested in fear, shame and silence. As I have shown, parents contribute to this discourse, as well as teachers. But the two participating teachers' claim of fear, as described earlier, is not groundless. Sexual violence and cases of HIV infection are prevalent in township contexts. Schools are not necessarily safe places, and parents know this. Township schools in South Africa are reported to have high levels of sexual abuse, and male teachers may sexually abuse and harass girls. Male teachers like Xaba who teach the Life Orientation curricula may find difficulty in dealing with and expressing opinions about sexuality in AIDS education because African males, including African male teachers, have been more generally demonised as sexual predators (Pattman & Bhana 2006). For Xaba, as a male teacher within a specific social context, his vulnerability to parental hostility is increased. If sexual speech is equated to sex, then this can be construed as sexual abuse.

To claim that talking about sex in AIDS education is bad information extends the claims that talking about sex is actually doing sex. Parental fears about schools and teachers with regard to sex and sexuality are not unjustifiable.

The circular power of fear (from parents and from teachers) increases anxiety about discussing sex. In contexts where there is high anxiety about the actual levels of sexual abuse of young children, and girls in particular (Richter *et al.* 2004), this fear is far from rhetorical.

At Bullwood, an overall ideal of childhood innocence was cushioned within the context of distancing from AIDS where talk about AIDS was not necessary and superseded by efforts to maintain the environment that supported innocence:

> Sing: They are very innocent . . . I think that parents . . . lots of the parents will object . . . I think that they are in a setting where they don't know much . . . So we don't talk too much about it. We don't say much about it. They just know it's a disease . . . and they don't talk about sex that much or at all . . . maybe it's old-fashioned but 'no.' . . . in class itself they don't get too much into it.
>
> Burke: I think it would need to [involve] calling parents in and discussing with them beforehand, there will be certain parents especially with—with certain religions that—that have a problem with discussing certain issues and—*ja*—so we would need a lot of parent support with it.

By foregrounding religion, Burke mediates knowledge about childhood inno-cence, parents and AIDS. A teacher's gaze on parents and religion, and thus on the children who inhabit this cultural world, will regulate and restrict the teaching of sexuality in AIDS education. Burke draws into a discourse in which teachers who talk with young people about sexuality may well find themselves the object of enquiry as they are seen to be promoting particular kinds of (undesirable) sexuality or encouraging children to become sexually active by introducing them to discussions about sexuality. This may com-promise their jobs and their identification as teachers in a primary school. Importantly, Burke focused on the possibility of partnerships with parents and their support in matters relating to sex and AIDS education. Despite the hegemony of childhood innocence, the possibilities do exist to disrupt the silence through working with parents. This results in a paradox between the need to maintain childhood innocence and the importance of addressing children as competent sexual actors.

Parents are diverse and the meanings they give to sex and AIDS education vary. However, it is necessary to note that because AIDS education involves discussing sex, working with parents around these issues will not always be easy. This is discussed in the next chapter.

## CONCLUSION

*Success in combating AIDS must be measured by its impact on chil-dren.* Are they getting the information they need to protect themselves from HIV? Are girls being empowered to take charge of their sexuality? These are hard questions we need to be asking . . .

—UNICEF (2002: 67)

In South Africa there is an unprecedented boom in sexual representation to include sexually explicit billboards suggesting safe sex and the dispensing of free condoms. The increased sexual momentum, underpinned by safer sex messages and instructions, on one hand, and the reality of young chil-dren's lives, on the other, coexists uneasily with teaching discourses attempt-ing to shut down sexual knowledge. There is a danger that the sinister allies—gender inequalities, AIDS and the romanticised notion of childhood innocence—will harm children, if not now then later (Bhana *et al.* 2006: 19). Talk about AIDS and sex as the teachers in this study illustrate, incited omi-nous fantasies, silence, danger, denial and shame.

Yet there is the implicit assumption throughout these teachers' construc-tions that young children are indeed sexual beings in their framing of AIDS education around warnings about the dangers of having sex. The notion of childhood innocence, as I have illustrated in this chapter, is not only formi-dable but is also resisted and reversible. The claim that children are young and innocent contrasts with Sishi's comment that "they already know". So we need to ask, now, about the potential of undermining the power of innocence. New understandings of children as active sexual agents (claimed by teachers even if contradictorily) make it necessary to reimagine the role of the teacher. Instead of attempting to privilege the notion of children's innocence, teachers might begin reworking dangerous narratives based on developmental approaches, which encourage a 'hands-off' approach to children's sexuality and their gender performance. It might be possible for teachers to intervene in creating opportunities in the new revised curriculum to raise critical and 'hard' questions about the sex, gender and AIDS relationships.

> The image of the child as innocent is highly exploitable by adults. In this study the social realities that mark the daily existence of young children is ignored through the construction of sexuality in AIDS education as undesirable. We need to begin to redefine childhood in ways that meet with the actual demands of the South African reality. We need to think of an image of childhood in which innocence and a need for protection do not depend on the renouncing of sexual understanding:
>     We've not even taught our children the very basic. And I feel that we have tried ignorance for a very long time and it's time we tried education.
>
> (Irvine, 2002: 1)

## REFERENCES

Baxen, J. and Breidlid, A. (Eds.) (2009). *HIV/AIDS in Sub-Saharan Africa. Understanding the Implications of Culture and Context*. Cape Town: UCT Press.

Bhana, D. (2006) 'The (Im)Possibility of Child Sexual Rights in Young South African Children's Account of HIV/AIDS'. *IDS Bulletin*, 37(4): 64–68.

Boyce, P., Huang Soo Lee, M., Jenkins, C., Mohamed, S., Overs, C., Paiva, V. & Aggleton, P. (2007) 'Putting Sexuality (Back) Into HIV/AIDS: Issues, Theory and Practice 1'. *Global Public Health*, 2(1): 1–34.

Campbell, C. (2003) *Letting Them Die: Why HIV/AIDS Intervention Programmes Fail*. Oxford: James Curry.

Department of Education (South Africa) (2005) *The Rights and Responsibilities of Parents, Learners and Public Schools*. Pretoria, Department of Education.

Epstein, D. & Johnson, R. (1998) *Schooling Sexualities*. Buckingham: Open University Press.

Francis, D.A. (2012) 'Teacher Positioning on the Teaching of Sexual Diversity in South African Schools'. *Culture, Health & Sexuality*, 14(6): 69–76.

Fuss, D. (1989) *Essentially Speaking: Feminism, Nature and Difference*. New York: Routledge.

Heinze, E. (ed) (2000) *Of Innocence and Autonomy Children, Sex and Human Rights*. Aldershot: Ashgate.

Human Rights Watch. (2001) *Scared at School: Sexual Violence Against Girls in South African Schools*. New York: Human Rights Watch.

Hunter, M. (2010) *Love in the Time of AIDS: Inequality, Gender, and Rights in South Africa*. Bloomington: Indiana University Press.

Irvine, J. M. (2002) *Talk About Sex: The Battles Over Sex Education in the United States*. Berkeley: University of California Press.

Iyer, P. & Aggleton, P. (2013) ' "Sexuality Education Should be Taught, Fine . . . But We Make Sure They Control Themselves": Teachers' Beliefs and Attitudes towards Young People's Sexual and Reproductive Health in a Ugandan Secondary School'. *Sex Education*, 13(1): 40–53.

Janssen, D. F. (2002) *Growing Up Sexually (Interim Report), October 2002. Volume 2: The Sexual Curriculum: The Manufacture and Performance of Pre-Adult Sexualities*. Amsterdam. Available online: http://www2.hu-berlin.de/sexology/ GESUND/ARCHIV/GUS/INDEX.HTM.

Kincaid, J. (1994) *Child Loving: The Erotic Child and Victorian Culture*. New York: Routledge.

MacNaughton, G. (2000) *Rethinking Gender in Early Childhood Education*. London: Paul Chapman Publishing.

Mayall, B. (2002) *Towards a Sociology of Childhood: Thinking from Children's Lives*. Buckingham: Open University Press.

Mellor, J. D. & Epstein, D. (2006) 'Sexualities and Schooling', in C. Skelton, B. Francis, & L. Smulyan (eds) *Handbook of Gender and Education* (pp. 378–391). Thousand Oaks, CA: Sage.

Miedema, E., Maxwell, C. & Aggleton, P. (2015) 'The Unfinished Nature of Rights Informed HIV- and AIDS-Related Education: An Analysis of Three School-Based Initiatives'. *Sex Education: Sexuality, Society and Learning*, 15(1): 78–92.

Morrell, R., Epstein D., Unterhalter, E., Bhana, D. & Moletsane, R. (2009). *Towards Gender Equality? South African Schools During the HIV/AIDS Epidemic*. Pietermaritzburg: University of KwaZulu-Natal Press.

Namisi, F. S., Flisher, A. J., Overland, S., Bastien, S., Onya, H., Kaaya, S. & Aarø, L. E. (2009) 'Socio-Demographic Variations in Communication on Sexuality and HIV/ AIDS With Parents, Family Members and Teachers among in School-Adolescents: A Multi-Site Study in Tanzania and South Africa'. *Scandinavian Journal of Public Health*, 37: 65–74.

Pattman, R. & Bhana, D. (2006) 'Black Boys With Bad Reputations'. *Alternations*, 13(2): 252–272.

Pattman, R. & Chege, F. (2003) *Finding Our Voices: Gendered and Sexual Identities in HIV/AIDS Education*. Nairobi: UNICEF ESARO.

Pred, A. (2000) *Even in Sweden: Racisms, Racialised Spaces and the Popular Geographical Imagination*. Berkeley: University of California Press.

Renold, E. (2005) *Girls, Boys and Junior Sexualities*. London: Routledge/Falmer.

Richter, L. M., Dawes, A, & Higson-Smith, C. (eds). (2004) *Sexual Abuse of Young Children in Southern Africa*. Pretoria: HSRC Press.

Robinson, S. (2013) 'Regulating the Race: Aboriginal Children in Private European Homes in Colonial Australia'. *Journal of Australian Studies*, 37(3): 302–315.

Sears, J. (ed) (1992) *Sexuality and the Curriculum*. New York: Teachers College Press.

Silin, J. (1995) *Sex, Death and the Education of Children: Our Passion for Ignorance in the Age of AIDS*. New York: Teachers College Press.

Stone, N., Ingham, R., & Gibbins, K. (2013) 'Where do babies come from?' Barriers to early sexuality communication between parents and young children. *Sex Education*, 13(2): 228–240.

Thorne, B. (1993) *Gender Play: Girls and Boys in School*. New Brunswick, NJ: Rutgers University Press.

Tobin, J. (ed). (1997) *Making a Place for Pleasure in Early Childhood Education*. New Haven, CT: Yale University Press.

UNICEF (2002) *Young People and HIV/AIDS: Opportunity in Crisis* UNICEF. New York: UNICEF.

Walkerdine, V. (2004) 'Development Psychology and the Study of Childhood', in M. Kehily (ed) *An Introduction to Childhood Studies* (pp. 112–124). Buckingham: Open University Press.

Watney, S. (1991) 'School's Out', in D. Fuss (ed) *Inside/Out: Lesbian Theories, Gay Theories* (pp. 387–404). London: Routledge.

Wood, L & Rolleri, L. A. (2014) 'Designing an Effective Sexuality Education Control Themselves': Teachers' Beliefs and Attitudes towards Young People's Sexual and Curriculum for Schools: Lessons Gleaned From the South(ern) African Literature'. *Sex Education: Sexuality, Society and Learning*, 14(5): 525–542.

# 7 True for All Mothers? Normalising Childhood Innocence

[T]he issue of sex education has not been easy . . . As a frontline AIDS activist I assumed that I should be able to manage it. But as an African woman, with all the baggage of taboos regarding talking about sex, it proved the hardest of tasks. Actually, in talking to women from other cultures, from the most industrialised to the poorest ones, I have found this to be true for all mothers . . .

—Kaleeba (2004: 277)

In the context of AIDS, why is it the "hardest of tasks" for mothers, whether rich or poor, to manage their role in the sexual constitution of children's AIDS-related knowledge? In previous chapters, I have argued that AIDS produces a paradox between the need to maintain childhood innocence and the importance of addressing children as competent sexual actors. Through examining how mothers of seven- and eight-year-old learners at KwaDabeka and Bullwood manoeuvre between this paradoxical space, this chapter illuminates the discursive practices through which childhood innocence is regulated and access to sexual information is made taboo. When mothers talk about the high expectation of and the need for childhood innocence and protection, they reproduce entrenched ideas about sexual innocence and protection from sexual knowledge and danger (Renold 2005; Martin 2009; Davies & Robinson 2010; Egan 2013; Robinson 2013). The restriction of children's power to express, know, feel, think and act sexually is central to the regulation of childhood sexuality and the production of innocence. As I have argued throughout the book, childhood sexuality is centrally about power and about the ways in which power is regulated, shaped and mediated. It is argued that childhood innocence is counterproductive to AIDS education and prevention. The association between sex and AIDS is shut down, and childhood innocence is upheld whilst simultaneously embedded within and governed by discourses of children's protection and children's vulnerability. Children's gendered and sexual competencies are relegated and denied, and their agency eroded, reproducing adult–child relations of inequalities. Like Kaleeba (2004), in this chapter I show that childhood innocence and child protection discourses are "true for all mothers"—rich and poor, both in Bullwood and KwaDabeka preventing effective discussion of sex and AIDS.

Beyond what holds "true for all mothers" are the varying social and cultural processes through which childhood innocence and child protection discourses are situated. Childhood innocence and child protection have a context, and mothers' practices and approaches are socially embedded. The signature of childhood innocence, as articulated by mothers in both contexts is stamped by gender, race and class illustrating the gendered/sexual fault lines of the AIDS pandemic and the web of networks that are social, sexual and of historical making. These social processes, as I have argued in this book, shape as they are shaped by the meanings that people give to gender, childhood sexuality and AIDS education. At KwaDabeka, the social structures of inequality, gender asymmetries of power and rampant male violence produce particular practices related to protection of children from sexual danger in which young girls' sexualities are rendered particularly vulnerable to sexual risk and HIV. In this context of high risk, mothers' approach to deal with sexual danger and HIV is to focus on talking to their daughters about rape and practices associated from distancing from dangerous men and boys. At Bullwood, and in the context of racialised class divides and privilege, AIDS is constructed as the disease of the other. Unlike children at KwaDabeka, caught within the matrix of poverty, structural inequalities, HIV, masculinities and violence, children at Bullwood are considered to be overprotected within supportive family networks where distancing mechanisms operate. Showing how race, class and culture are deployed in upholding innocence, I contend in this chapter that childhood innocence is not simply a monolithic expression of power but is also embedded within the varying social contexts which make up the South African landscape. At Bullwood mothers' approaches to sexual socialisation are highly racialised and classed, reproducing childhood innocence and refracting it through AIDS as the disease of the other. As Silin (1995: 25) notes,

> [w]hen AIDS is viewed as the disease of the Other, it allows us to feel safe. The physical and emotional realities of the disease are not possibilities for our own lives and can be discounted. To give up this pose is to acknowledge that the possibility of the Other is also my possibility . . . We resist knowing the Other as if hoping that our ignorance will protect us, guaranteeing safety from infection.

This chapter shows both the continuities and the social and cultural variations in the way childhood innocence is caught up in mothers' approaches to and practices related to their role in the sexual socialisation of children's AIDS-related knowledge.

## KWADABEKA AND BULLWOOD MOTHERS: AIDS, SEX AND CONSTRUCTION OF CHILDHOOD INNOCENCE

Debates about power are central to the conceptualisation of child-hood innocence. The core of the issue is that children's socialisation, it is assumed, excludes (or de-emphasises) the possibility that children are sexual beings. In this conceptualisation of childhood innocence, children are seen as victims of sexuality and a prerogative of adult knowledge and power. This version of childhood innocence invests in and permits the reproduction of children as needing protection from sexuality, and ascribes adults and mothers in particular with power to do so. In this section mothers' shared approach to sexual socialisation in the children's AIDS-related knowledge draws on developmental stages of learning sexuality whilst displacing sexual knowledge to sexual abuse, danger and blood and contagion. Despite the wide variation in social experiences, mothers had shared views about their responsibility for their children's education and well-being. At KwaDabeka, mothers were overburdened by the context of father absence and what they termed "father irresponsibility" in providing and caring for families. At Bullwood, fathers were "busy" in powerful economic positions. The social and economic conditions were such that mothers were mainly the routine source of knowledge and information in the home:

> Ayanda: Today I am the one who takes care of everything . . . I am at home to help my mother because she is very old and I am the one to make sure my children have food and go to school. They talk to me and I have to answer the questions.
>
> Caroline: . . . '[C]ause life's busy, dads aren't even home sometimes when you sit down to do dinner, or like my husband's away two weeks out of every month . . . but I think in reality it's the mom more often than not.
>
> Sophie: I think moms just generally create a routine, that routine is also part of the safety and security, you kind of know what's gonna happen, it's not just chaos um, you eat when you're hungry or grab something and go and sit in front of the TV, you know, things are organised and life is planned . . . I think, I think the child needs to be secure at home and safe to be able to ask questions and make mistakes.

Even in the West the marginalisation of fathers' involvement in and mothers' established role in young children's health and education are noted (Davies & Robinson 2010). Mothers' investments in their own position as primary caregivers and critical in providing information about AIDS was shared although on matters of sex this was complex, drawing on a range of

discursive strategies invoking age, sexual abuse and contagion and producing childhood innocence and protection discourses:

> Bongile:   One day my boy asked where I got him from. When I told
> him that I bought him from the aeroplane, he asked me how
> he came from the plane to the hospital. He told me that
> I was lying and I could see that he knows about giving birth.
>
> Georgina:   I think at this young age, Kirsten [her seven-year-old
> daughter] is still watching *Cinderella* and she, she's al-
> ready talking about getting married, I mean she just wants
> to have the white dress and building on top of our house
> so she and her family can live upstairs and they can visit
> us downstairs [laughs].

Avoiding the facts of life about how children are conceived (see also Stone
*et al.* 2013) and constructing children's lives in relation to mythical and
magical sources of information and frivolous play point to regulatory strategies. Cinderella becomes the metaphor for innocence. The myths combined
with gendered and heterosexual futures are not separate from each other
and are configured in ways that interact dynamically with each other to
form a hegemonic version of childhood innocence. Children's worlds are
assumed to be pure and untainted by sexually corrupting knowledge. Yet,
as the preceding examples illustrate, children do know: "I could see that
he knows about giving birth". In the second transcript, the normalisation
of heterosexuality through an imagined future suggests that playing Cinderella and wearing a white dress are early stages of childhood sexuality
through which gender and heterosexuality are normalised (Martin 2009).
Heterosexuality (Martin 2009) is premised on everyday normative practices
that are seen as natural and are taken for granted. Georgina's focus on her
daughter Kirsten's interest in Cinderella is locked into what Butler (2004)
refers to as gender performativity, through which a heterosexual femininity is produced. Kelly's description suggests that instead of sexuality being
absent in children's lives, it is actively performed and embedded in the very
early stages of children's life although the taken-for-granted assumption of
heterosexuality is presumed and childhood innocence is locked into this
state of naturalisation. Mothers were defining and regulating what they
wished for (Epstein & Johnson 1998) in order to preserve a naturalised
image of sexual innocence.

Avoidance of sexual matters in AIDS-related knowledge also took the
excuse identified by Stone *et al.* (2013: 237), "if they don't ask, they don't
want to know and aren't ready to know".

> Kelly:   I've always waited for whatever questions they ask and then
> give them *ja*, give them the answer but not all the details just
> enough to suffice for that point . . . without sort of getting
> them too curious.

Waiting for children to ask discomforting sexual questions assumes that sexuality is not part of children's lives, and reproduces the idealisation of sexual purity and children's sexual knowledge as a taboo subject. In order to maintain the image of childhood innocence, sexual curiosity is avoided by limiting and regulating appropriate knowledge through age-appropriate information. The loss of childhood innocence was considered a major concern amongst all mothers and they did want to destroy innocence by giving too much of information:

> Caroline:   . . . [T]hat's destroying the innocence . . . and, *ja*. . that's taking the child away.

To reclaim the innocent child, mothers strategically advanced their roles as caring for and protecting children from sexually corrupt knowledge. Related to this strategy were concerns that sex could fuel sexual activity (and immorality):

> Dudu:   It's difficult for us as Africans to talk about sex to our children . . . what can I say . . . when you try to explain to your child about sex, it's as if, you as a parent is teaching your child to be immoral. That's why I say it's difficult to be exact, but we try our best to warn them about AIDS.
> Mbali:   We are afraid that we will be encouraging our children to go out there and experience if we talk about it.

It is assumed that talk about sex provokes sexual experience. By implication not talking about sex, protects the innocence of children against the corruption of sexuality. Instead of conceptualising sexuality as central to childhood, an essentialist account of the child is hegemonised. Contradictorily, there is nothing natural about childhood innocence because of the fear that children can be transformed into sexual beings if sex was talked about. In other words, sexuality can be denied, hidden and silenced when not spoken about. However, mothers did not see this as a denial of childhood sexuality; rather, not talking about it was part of the overall strategy to avoid sensitive matters with children, to increase the children's risk anxiety and to negotiate the mothers' power and their discomfort in addressing childhood sexuality. An appeal to essentialist versions of childhood and race become apparent when Dudu states, "For us as Africans", as if there is something innate in African conceptualisations of childhood and sex.

Age and age-appropriate debates were central to mothers' shared narratives of childhood innocence. There was much debate about and anxieties concerning the age at which children were rightfully equipped to deal with the sexual part of AIDS-related information. Some mothers suggested that age-appropriate knowledge was 10, others vacillated between 11 and 15 years. Drawing from developmental theory, older children were assumed to have better skills in understanding sexuality whilst others considered the end of primary school (ages 12 to 13 years) or the beginning of high school as more appropriate. Critical in this debate about the age at which young children should be informed of sex and AIDS was the mothers' anxieties about transgressing childhood innocence. Whilst all mothers agreed that their children had to learn about sex and AIDS-related knowledge, the common discourse 'too young to know' prevailed:

> Busi:    . . . [I]t's better to talk to a 15-year-old because may be they will understand what I am talking about. I just tell myself that 15 will be the time when she will understand things better . . .
>
> Jabu:    I know that I have to talk to him because there is no use of keeping these things a secret. But I will wait until he is ten . . .
>
> Kelly:   Well, they've gotta get out there sooner or later so they've gotta be equipped . . . sort of late primary school and high school.
>
> Amy:     *Ja*, senior primary they did, grade 5 I think . . .
>
> Abby:    I'm confused, um, 10, 11 rather.
>
> Amy:     They're already starting periods at nine, ten, the little girls so *ja*, nine or ten.

The discussion about the appropriate age at which to discuss sex in AIDS-related knowledge was linked to the deep anxiety that mothers felt in violating childhood innocence that needed to be protected. Drawing from developmental theory and ages and stages of development, access to sexual knowledge at seven and eight years of age could be deleterious for children. Sexuality was viewed as an abstract issue, but as Amy notes earlier, access to sexual knowledge could also be based when girls began menstruating, which also suggested a narrow biological version of sexual knowledge (Bennett & Harden 2014).

> Amy:     I haven't used the um, technical terms which you probably should do but I said you've got three holes; one, one for stinkers, [all laugh] one for wees and one for babies to come out and that's just what happens . . . and that's enough for her to know at that point and she's actually, I think, she's too shy to ask anything.

If children are too shy to ask, admittedly they know already by age seven that sexuality is aligned to secrets, silences and taboos. Mothers' responses to sexual questions—"too soon to tell" and "answer only if asked"—avoid anatomical terms, deploying euphemisms suggest how sexuality is shameful and answer within limits without transgressing the illusory laws of innocence.

When it came to discussions about what mothers taught their children concerning AIDS, blood and contagion featured prominently in their approach and practices to children's AIDS-related knowledge, which functioned strategically to displace sex:

Amy:      . . . [T]hey definitely seem to, to pick up very early on the idea that, that blood can be infected and um, that's the main thing actually at this age, . . . that's the risk that they face is touching other people's blood, at this age.

Caroline:  I think the basic of AIDS, of, infected blood . . . I mean the kids are on the playground, they need to know that from an early age but I think the sex side of things that needs to be sort of done very sort of, just as a matter of fact sort of, until they're a bit older, because it takes away the kids part that suddenly they're suddenly aware of themselves and not just letting themselves go and just running around in the garden and all that sort of thing so it's, it's, I don't know, it's hard. . .

Ayanda:   . . . I know that we must tell our children about HIV . . . like I tell my daughter that if anyone gets hurt at school and bleed, she is not supposed to touch anybody's blood . . . she mustn't touch blood. I tell her that if she touches somebody else's blood she will have a problem, AIDS.

The easiest way through which knowledge of AIDS was imparted was through the AIDS and blood equation. Blood induced a sense of fear and triggered contagion, but it had a far more strategic value. The focus on blood allowed mothers to deny, silence and hide knowledge about sexual matters. Understanding AIDS through blood and contagion was considered age appropriate, not sex.

On the question of sex, sexual abuse and danger received priority. Sexuality is constituted through a framework that positioned children as vulnerable, helpless and potential victims of sexual abuse consistent with other research (Renold 2005; Robinson 2013). Whilst children were regarded as incompetent to understand and express sexuality, the contradiction here is that children are capable of understanding their bodies and the privacy only in relation to bad touches and in relation to "people who might want to hurt them":

Caroline:  . . . [Y]ou teach them about their bodies, that their bodies are private, that only certain people like doctors and their parents are allowed to touch them in, in private areas and I think maybe that's the start at this age, and you don't want to scare them but you have to alert them to the fact that sometimes people aren't always there to be kind to you, sometimes there are people who might want to hurt them . . .

Yoking childhood innocence and sexual danger created overwhelming anxiety, and the protection of children from sexual predators was a tremendous concern across the sites. Protection from sexual predators reinforced childhood innocence. Sexual purity is set up against sexual abuse. Kitzinger

(1998) calls this the theft of innocence. Kitzinger notes that children are rendered helpless victims and vulnerable without power to ward off sexual danger. Silin (1995: 199) writes that "the innocent child is always ignorant, empty of knowledge, in need of protection: the perfect receptacle for the adult's imaginings". The emphasis on sexual abuse reproduces the idea of children's incompetency with regard to sexual expression and their immunity to sexuality whilst reproducing their exotic status as pure and innocent. Mothers were very aware of their responsibilities towards their children regarding sexual matters, but such responsibility was clearly gendered because girls' sexuality needed greater protection:

> Lungile:  I tell her about not letting anyone touch her private parts and if there is anyone who does that to her, she must report to the teachers or to me.
>
> Buhle:    I talk to her but it's difficult. In actual fact we know that we must talk to our children about sex as we know what is happening outside there. What if there is someone who touches my child where she is not supposed to be touched, her private part and then she keeps quiet and does not report to me because I did not talk about this to her? I think we have to talk to them about rape. I say do not allow any person to touch your private part and do not to accept any money or gifts from strangers or talk to them.

In the context where innocence is highly sexualised, it is also highly gendered (Kincaid 1998; Renold 2005). As the next section shows, girls' vulnerability to rape and HIV is a serious concern, but the main point here is that mothers at both sites were concerned primarily with the protection of girls' innocence.

## KWADABEKA MOTHERS AND CHILD PROTECTION: AIDS, RAPE, POVERTY AND THE SCANDAL OF MANHOOD

How do child protection discourses gain a foothold in the mothers' approaches and practices to children's AIDS-related knowledge? When mothers speak of their role in the sexual socialisation of children's AIDS-related knowledge, they do not talk from a blank page. Their approaches and practices are rooted within social, economic, cultural and ideological contexts, underscoring the contextual basis of childhood innocence and child protection. By focusing on African mothers emerging from and overburdened by conditions of chronic poverty, underwritten by apartheid, gender inequalities, living precarious lives and relying on social grants, this section gives priority to mothers' objection to and critique of an 'irresponsible' and toxic masculinity and the contradictory contours of power which shape and influence their practices in relation AIDS education and to the sexual constitution of children. Mothers' narratives operate along a continuum and are enmeshed within social and cultural conditions, which create vulnerability for children and girls at KwaDabeka, (as Chapter 4 has demonstrated), as it does for women. These social conditions are also the primary culprits behind women and girls' disproportionate vulnerability to sexual violence and HIV. A central argument in this section is that the mothers' approach to child protection, and the protection of girls in particular, is not as passive victims of structural and social inequalities. Their practices take place in a context of limited options and poor support. Their approach to the sexual constitution of their children to AIDS-related knowledge both challenges and reproduces vulnerability.

First, mothers discussed the context of grinding poverty, food scarcity, unemployment and the inability of men and fathers to provide:

Cebile:   I struggle by myself to bring up my children because their father doesn't have money . . .

Lungile:   Men do not support their families. They are not serious about looking for jobs and the money they get from the temporary jobs they use it to buy alcohol.

Buhle:   When I grew up . . . I grew up believing that it's my father who was supporting the family, but when I think carefully about it now, it was my mother who was the backbone of my family. Even today men are like that, they don't support their families . . . being irresponsible.

Unemployment is a key development problem in South Africa (Bernstein 2014) and is deeply intertwined with male power and weakness. The inability of men to provide must be situated within broader expressions of masculinity in KwaZulu-Natal, where the cultural ideals of fatherhood correlates with breadwinning status and the ability to build a home, take care of and provide for a family (Hunter 2010; Bhana & Nkani 2014). The conversations with mothers show how the dynamics of male unemployment and male irresponsibility locks into the everyday suffering, food scarcity and men's lack of care in families. Unemployment and male frailty in achieving breadwinning status crystallises into male weakness and struggle for women albeit as the "backbone of the family". Fathers and men do not have monolithic power. As I have argued in previous chapters, the structural inequalities have historical and economic origins and are changing, but these inequalities have effects on women and children most marginalised by the political economy. The linkage between male unemployment, the lack of care and contribution to families, power and sexual violence is complex but has a deep-rooted effect on the mothers' construction of child protection discourses. Whilst African men have historically been seen as providers, their inability to do so has meant that the mothers' role as contributors and carers is highlighted:

> Jabu:    What I do is to look for temp [temporary domestic work] in order to buy whatever we need at home . . . and pay school fees . . . I try by all means to spend their [child support grant] money on them . . . if I don't provide . . . they will accept money and gifts from strangers or go to our neighbours . . . They could end up being raped . . . They can be easily enticed by money from men and end up being hurt . . . Most of the time those men who rape children entice them with money or sweets. They say, "Come here, I'll give money . . ."

The child support grant, whilst meagre is meaningful in a context where the material basis of sexual relations and coercive sexual practices is clear. At the nexus of poverty and domination, mothers' resourcefulness derives from access to the social grant system compensating for dire poverty, as well as their efforts to obtain temporary work to alleviate children's economic distress and vulnerability to coercive sexual relations. The materiality of sexual coercion is established, and girls' vulnerability to transactional relations is manifest very early in life. Hunter (2006) and Silberschmidt (2001) suggest African men's economic inability to achieve successful masculinity in building a home has produced disempowerment and could explain why men abandon their families and use violence/sexual violence to re-establish lost power which mothers identify as "irresponsibility". When mother's talk about child protection, they talk about acute gendered inequalities, unemployment, male violence and poverty, and these come together to explain the social context of child protection at KwaDabeka.

Women's overburdened social conditions were exacerbated by male alcohol abuse and the horror of sexual and gender violence limiting the exercise of power:

> Buhle:    They [men] are very irresponsible. Sometimes they don't even come home to check whether you have anything to eat. Even if they have piece [temporary] jobs, they'll buy drink with all that money, come home drunk . . . demand food. They then fight with everybody at home. The children cannot go to sleep because he is fighting with them and they even hide under the table. They are no longer happy to see their father he has become a monster to them . . . like when he comes home the children feel like hiding. I am also afraid of him because he beats me . . .

Living at the very bottom of the social ranks, mothers situate their role in facilitating the sexual socialisation of their children's AIDS-related knowledge within the horror of fear and violence perpetrated by men in the home which has an impact on the most marginalised—the women and children—thus constraining agency. Children "hide" from violent fathers and mothers are "afraid". When I asked Buhle why she stayed with her husband she said, "I still love him". Economic misery combined with gender norms and affection creates vulnerabilities, which materialise into relations of domination and subordination where women's agency is diminished. In this crucible of unemployment, food insecurity, gender violence and male entitlements, the mothers' endorsement of child protection is given its appropriate context of interpretation.

Next, mothers focused on the scandal of masculinity as it related to multiple partners and sexual entitlements:

Busi:   Many women are beaten by their husbands, and if they refuse to sleep with them. Some are even chased out of their homes because of refusing to sleep with their husbands and are locked outside.

As Jewkes *et al.* (2014) argue, intimate partner relations, gender and cultural norms, male sexual entitlements, poverty and inequality coalesce to reduce women's and girls' ability to negotiate safe sex:

Fikile:   Men are the ones who are spreading AIDS because . . . he doesn't remain faithful to his partner. He continues with his many affairs spreading AIDS. Sometimes he gets drunk and has sex without using a condom and when he goes for [a] test he will find himself positive. Sometimes he doesn't even bother to take the test.

Lungile:   My boyfriend pretends as if he is working on weekends and he sleeps with other women. When I ask him whether he is not afraid of AIDS he will tell me that he doesn't mind dying because of sex because he was made through sex.

Buhle:   . . . [M]y husband too pretends as if he is going to work whereas he is visiting his girlfriends and comes back with AIDS. I am no longer feeling free to be with him.

The question of sexual socialisation of children and AIDS-related knowledge is enmeshed within complex social forces invoking sexuality, gender relations of power, masculinity and race/class. Whilst mothers talked about fathers who could not provide, they also talked pervasively about a sexually irresponsible masculinity where men who do not test for HIV status nor do they protect themselves or their partners against HIV. Combined with male violence against women and reckless sexuality, the fear of men and sexual danger looms large in the everyday life at KwaDabeka, squeezing women and girls' agency. The mothers' role in facilitating children's sexual literacy in AIDS-related knowledge must be situated under social conditions which are both inimical to children's and mothers' well-being and hostile to gender equality.

In bringing these co-factors together in understanding the social context of children's lives, mothers' approach and practice to children's AIDS-related knowledge is to childhood sexuality within a protectionist discourse. Within this framing it is girls who are rendered vulnerable to and victims of rape. These are continuities between mothers' own experiences and their knowledge of rape in the community. Indeed, mothers noted that they were afraid of the violence of men, accused men of spreading HIV and objected to men who "don't respect women" and rape. Posel (2005: 127) notes that in the context of AIDS in South Africa, "it is the very intimacy of the home—mother, father and children—which has become contaminated. And it is men particularly—the fathers and sons of the nation—whose moral credibility is most acutely called into question."

For mothers at KwaDabeka, AIDS becomes the metaphor for rape, the terror of sexual violence, where the fear of boys and men heightens the need for child protection:

> Busi:    They [children] are raped by even their fathers, stepfathers, uncles, neighbours even by strangers, but they are mostly raped by their relatives and children are mostly raped by the people they know. That is why we teach them that they must be afraid of men, uncle, brother or a neighbour even before it happens to your own child. You tell them that if any man calls her, she must tell him that my mother told me not to come near you if she is not around.

Contextual dimensions of mothers approach to children's AIDS-related knowledge and practice are embedded within an environment hostile to gender equality and where girls' are vulnerable to rape:

> Fikile:    AIDS is not going away . . . it is not going to disappear . . . so we must talk about it to our children. We must talk about it . . . like me, I talk to Thobeka [her daughter] . . . I don't actually talk about sex, I only tell her not to be too friendly with boys like when you play, play only with other girls. I know that there are boys at school, she can play with them in the classroom, but out of the classroom I tell her to play with girls only.
>
> Busi:    I tell them that they mustn't go near girls because if they do so they'll be taken to jail . . . I'm afraid of talking about sex with them. They are still young . . . I only say, "Do not go near girls".

As discussed in Chapter 6, the approach and practice to children's AIDS-related knowledge is to situate sexuality within the domain of fear and danger to restrict sexual matters. Mothers adopted similar strategies. Boys and girls are polarised because their relationships are assumed to be unavoidably sexual and dangerous. Sex is considered the source of connection between boys and girls. Child protection implies separation of boys and girls and girls from men. Pattman (2005) argues that the polarisation of boys from girls is unlikely to end sexual violence and works to reinforce girls as weak and without any capacity to reflect, act and work on their circumstances. It is also important to address what the polarisation creates for boys who are regarded as potentially sexually dangerous in relation to girls.

## BULLWOOD MOTHERS AND CHILDHOOD INNOCENCE: AIDS, RACE, CLASS AND OTHERNESS

In contrast to KwaDabeka mothers whose narratives bears the mark of children's vulnerability in the crucible of violence and deep rooted social inequalities, Bullwood mothers' approaches and practices in addressing the sexual constitution of children's AIDS related knowledge were premised on overprotection:

> Sophie: . . . I suppose we're lucky because our children are actually very protected, particularly us who work from home or who are available for our kids. We pick them ourselves from school, we're there with them all afternoon, our children are never where they're not safe . . . so I think for us AIDS is not as big an issue. You know our children don't have to walk to and from school, they don't have to, have to go in a, in a, like, public transport, they're not left on their own at home or in some aftercare that you don't know the people running it. I think that's difficult for us to actually put our heads around it because we don't actually face the same problems as other parents probably do.
>
> Caroline: Yes, you know, our children are actually very lucky, they're actually almost *overprotected* in a way because, *ja*, I agree, I don't think AIDS for us is a big issue . . . At such a young age, *ja*, there are other things . . . [emphasis added].

Like the mothers at KwaDabeka, the mothers at Bullwood talk from a social and economic context producing an approach that upholds childhood innocence. Like the mothers at KwaDabeka, the mothers at Bullwood do not work, but their life experiences and narratives are intertwined with economic capital and male success on the economic front and bear the signature of historical privilege and power, leading to the construction of their children as "lucky" and "overprotected". The differential distribution of power between mothers at KwaDabeka and Bullwood is clear, and this power is mobilised to create difference and separation from the problems of AIDS, "because we don't actually face the same problems as other parents probably do". Living in a context of material abundance and plentiful resources, "overprotection" is the effect of racial privilege, the history of apartheid and the context in which vulnerability to HIV is substantially reduced. Mothers' approach to children and their practices were premised on time spent with their children, protection, care and support reproducing familiar notions of intensive mothering practices associated with middle class white women (Kawash 2011; O'Reilly 2006). For the mothers at Bullwood, mothering was associated with presence and was deeply embedded within their historically privileged social and economic status. This permitted their status as "stay-at-home moms" and allowed access to good schooling for their children. Within this nexus of privilege, the possibilities for feminist commitment to, and in their approach to, children were also evident:

> Abby:      I treat my girls um, as I, as I would have treated boys and, and not limit them in, in any way, you know, make them believe that they can be whatever they want to be, you know.
>
> Caroline:  Both my boys know how to do a basic meal, if I'm not around they can boil an egg, they can make toast, they both know how to make tea and all that sort of thing, . . . I know that they are quite capable of doing things and they do chores . . . there's no such thing in our house that because it, it's a girl thing or a boy thing. If things are to be done then that's what it's gotta be.

The standards of good mothering include feminist-orientated principles, but these are dependent on the combination of social factors elucidated earlier. The question of mothers' role in facilitating children's AIDS-related sexual knowledge runs deep and wide into the social and economic contexts that imprint their particular practices. Childhood innocence at Bullwood is driven by a combination of privilege, low infection rates amongst white South Africans, a turn to gender-equitable relationships, stable family life and distancing from the problem of AIDS. In a context where children navigate "safe" zones the mothers' approach AIDS education as "not a big issue, at such a young age". The aggregate effects of race, class, gender and histories of privilege mean that mothers' approach their children's knowledge of AIDS with reduced perceptions of vulnerability, an issue of diminished relevance and where age combines to produce sexual silence.

"Not a big issue, at such a young age" does not take place in a vacuum. It combines social, economic and political ideologies, mobilised by racialised histories in South Africa to reproduce a version of childhood as untainted and unaffected by the problems of others—in this instance, the problem of crime and AIDS in the country is the problem with Africans:

> Sophie:   At this young age, I think Kayla [daughter], um, you, you're right, um, more, Kayla is more worried about a robber getting into our house. Have I locked the doors, did I lock the boot?

> Even the boot, somebody had told her a story, their mother's bag was stolen out the boot . . . that kind of thing so I think the crime at this age is more of a worry, I mean, . . . It's more in your face . . .

Amy:   I actually volunteer at the Hillcrest AIDS Centre on a Monday and a Tuesday, I help with the feeding scheme, and *ja*, particularly the Zulu culture and those women, for them to try and break out of that mould is so difficult because it's been bred into them that they are subservient, and if their husband goes away and sleeps with a whole lot of different women, they just have to accept that, they can't fight back and *ja*, it's I think we've got a huge fight on our hands with that.

Alex:   I think more of worry is, um, the crime statistics than being, being, become HIV, and that is a big worry here because it seems to be, a, whether it's a cultural thing to have the power over females or whether it's a thing coming from a witchdoctor that if you rape a white woman you, or a woman, or a virgin, or a child or a something, you're cured, you know there's a lot of that goes on in the culture and that I think is, almost more of a fear . . . in being raped and then being, being, HIV, and that is a big worry here. . .

The mothers' discussions about HIV reveal deeper pathologies of power (Farmer 2006). Material and social structures of inequality have created a context in South Africa, where crime and violence are manifestations of stark inequalities for the majority African working class in the context of deep poverty where their vulnerability to AIDS is increased. When mothers talk about crime and AIDS, it triggers an us/them logic based on the good and evil, the innocent and savage and the vulnerable, fuelling child protection (Silin 1995). Both crime and AIDS strongly reinforces the distancing from and the reinforcement of Africans as perpetrators of violence, crime and vectors in the spread of the disease. In this equation, African men and culture are pathologised, and the racist equation becomes apparent. In doing so mothers construct race through culturally degenerate practices—of African men—that involve rape and child rape, gender inequalities, women's subordination and white women's own vulnerability to HIV through rape. In other words, African men are diseased vectors in the spread of the disease disrupting the stability of middle class families, leading to "worry". As McClintock (1995) argues, racialised tropes on African sexuality construct the African male sexual predator and the exotic construction of sexuality in racialised ways that fuel white fear and white women's particular risk (Stoller 2002). AIDS comes to Bullwood only in the context of African criminal masculinity reproducing racist chasms (Petros *et al.* 2006).

AIDS as a contaminating force was also brought into the civilised world of Bullwood when mothers referred to mixed-race/-class schools and domestic workers in their homes:

> Amy:      [I]t's a cultural thing, because you've got black children in the school who are exposed to so much more themselves so it's the norm for them to see a couple having sex, you know, because they share rooms and things, depending on where they, they live, which your own children are not being exposed to but it's all spoken about and it's just the norm at school.
>
> Sophie:   I also think where there are maids working in a home, if the maid has lost a child through AIDS or whatever and the topic comes up that would, it would bring it up, um, and also, and staff, you know, any of the staff at school have passed, passed away . . . and I think um, with bussing in children . . .
>
> Karen:    . . . [T]hey showed on TV this morning in the Eastern Cape, nine people living in this one-roomed shack. They're worried about the cold and all that, and the one has got, got AIDS and having to have medication and they don't even have blankets and, you know, just implications, you know, one does go to school. Now you can just imagine what he's telling his friends his about his home environment, so it's going to . . . because of the integrated school system you're going to hear more stories.

When AIDS comes to Bullwood, it links race and class, poor and rich and invokes the construction of a racialised, diseased and contaminated other. AIDS at Bullwood is considered out of context. Race is socially constructed but has real material and discursive consequences in relation to the social construction of gender and African sexuality. Race and AIDS are tied together so that the African other is potentially threatening to the sanitised middle-class/elite white context. Whilst media reports of suffering related to AIDS and poverty produce a context of pity, when AIDS comes to close to Bullwood, it is racialised, othered and feared. AIDS is presented to Bullwood in the context of desegregating classrooms and where increasing numbers of African learners attend formerly all-white schools, through "bussing", and this produces the terror of AIDS. In the home of middle class families, AIDS enters the home through domestic worker narratives of AIDS-related deaths. Whilst AIDS is regarded as peripheral, the pandemic is a striking reminder of the social network that links Bullwood and KwaDabeka, poverty and plenty, in ways that reproduce and challenge the social processes through which childhood innocence is constructed. Childhood innocence is mobilised through fear and distancing and through the construction of race and class inequalities. However, contradictions emerged. As mothers reflected on the sexual socialisation of their older children and examples of HIV amongst white South Africans and white vulnerability to disease:

> Sophie:   Yes, I have a huge fear . . . I have a friend that I was at school with from primary school to Matric. He was, um, considered in those days as the nerd, he didn't play the rugby and cricket, he was into chess and photography and that type thing so had never had a girlfriend, and after the army, um, moved into digs with a couple of guys and they would have their parties. He on a one-night stand got AIDS and he today . . . he's been boarded from work because he's always tired and can't keep up and he has met a woman um, who's also got AIDS, from England . . . and he can't go and live there and you know it's just, and he's only 42 . . . if it was my son, *ja*, it would be a dependent forever, it's like having a physically disabled child, you are, that child is dependent on you forever but it could've been prevented and then start looking at yourself and saying why didn't, what did I do or what didn't I do? I would feel responsible because it's like giving a child a death sentence, I don't know, I just . . .

AIDS is socially produced. It is not as distant as previously discussed by mothers. The knowledge of infection in a middle-class white context does open questions about responsibility and about how to address prevention:

> Abby:   We don't like to think about it, let's be honest, none of us do, we like to think that it's 'their' disease but it's, *ja*.
>
> Kelly:   But the incidents, I think are isolated, that we hear about, you know, children like ours getting infected.

Importantly, what is regarded as the disease of the 'other' can no longer be sustained. The us/them logic is broken down, but Kelly is quick to ensure that the incidents are isolated and reverts to the dominant discourse through which AIDS is racialised.

The contradiction also emerged in relation to mothers' reflection of children's sexual socialisation, although this too was framed alongside danger:

> Victoria:   . . . I am more concerned about my daughter and it's also a perception, it's not gonna happen to me and that's what we have to get through to our children . . . yes, it does happen to white children from good homes, decent schools, it does, it happen to everybody, it only takes once . . . one . . . silly sexual encounter, you know, that's all it takes.
>
> Barbara:   I just think that the way the world is and the way, the dangers our children actually face, you actually can't afford to be shy and namby-pamby about it, you actually can't.

Abby:      . . . [Y]ou don't want them hearing things from other kids at school because you don't know what they're being told. I feel it's much better coming from you as a parent than to hear things and then they might hear horrible things that they are now too scared to talk to you about it, so . . .

Camilla:   Well, the bottom line is, you are their role model . . . and you've gotta give the right information, sort of thing that they can, and you're a safety net as well . . . coming home is a safety net, you both have got to feel secure and safe . . . it's, basically, bottom-line is that you are the kid's safety net so you've gotta be able to talk to them and be with them and, and deal with whatever . . . that's troubling them.

AIDS, Silin (1995) notes, is a disease of contradictions. Beyond the racialised construction of the disease, are the contradictions that AIDS does happen to white people and that a "silly sexual encounter" can be the basis to take action. AIDS does present a moment when mothers at Bullwood can reflect on and consider the prospects of changing familiar practices with children especially because the stakes are high. AIDS-related knowledge and the education of children, in the final analysis, are the responsibility of parents, as is providing the right information—"you are the kid's safety net so you've gotta be able to talk to them".

## CONCLUSION

Why is it the "hardest of tasks" for mothers, whether rich or poor, is to manage their role in the sexual socialisation of children's AIDS-related knowledge? This chapter has been concerned with exploring mothers' approach to and practices in the sexual socialisation of children's AIDS-related knowledge. The chapter draws attention to the ways in which childhood innocence and child protection is socially constructed and mediated by race and class. Mothers' approaches and practices are embedded in and governed by the need to shut down sex in AIDS-related education. Yet, as I have claimed in this book, the AIDS paradox presents childhood innocence and child protection alongside the need to address children as agents with capacity to reflect on, filter through, act on and make sense of sexual and gender issues. It is within this paradoxical nexus that mothers negotiate, mediate and struggle as their produce childhood innocence. Mothers were united in their support for children's AIDS-related education, but how, what and the extent to which they could draw on the sexual remained controversial mobilised by their ambivalence towards sexual decadence and excess sexual knowledge which they believed could defile childhood.

In this chapter I identified the various discursive strategies through which mothers legitimated the sanitisation of AIDS-related knowledge. Mothers were united in their positions as primary caregivers and principally responsible for children's health, well-being and education (Martin 2009). I describe how mothers' approaches to reproduction, age, blood, contagion and sexual abuse are complexly intertwined. They are interdependent and mutually constructing, forming an overall strategy that regulates and casts children as unprotesting victims of sexuality, without power and at risk to sexual abuse (Egan & Hawkes 2009). In the context of grave concerns related to sexual violence against children in South Africa, there are real dangers that children face as they navigate their social worlds. Like Jackson and Scott (2010) I do not share the agenda of Furedi (2006): that fears or risk are social imaginings premised on a 'culture of fear'. Real dangers threaten South African society and call into question the specific social conditions which produce children's vulnerability to sexual danger and girls' vulnerability to HIV. However, I seriously question the conservative and hegemonic patterns through which mothers approach childhood sexuality. It is not knowledge of sexuality that endangers children. How not to talk about sex, how to avoid it and how to displace sex from AIDS education does not promote children's sexual health and well-being. Ironically, mothers concerns about sexual danger and harm are actually bred in the home, in a context in which there is reluctance, even misinformation, in being honest about sex and AIDS. Denial, silence and misplacement are previously positioned children's safety as the illusory ideal of childhood innocence is pursued. Indeed withholding information about sex and sexuality in AIDS-related education cannot be endorsed and work against the articulation and practices of children's right to knowledge and information that is key to their safety, health and well-being. Children are placed at risk of developing sexual and gendered behaviours that might produce vulnerability to HIV and other sexual risks if not now, then in the future. It is vital for mothers who are themselves invested in their critical caregiving roles to understand that honesty about sex in AIDS-related knowledge might increase children's competency, enable open and honest discussion with children and allow them the right to express, ask questions, laugh and debate about the issues as they have done with me. Chapters 2, 3, and 4 show how competent children are as gendered and sexual beings, powerful, protesting, desiring, interested as they mediate and confront the mockery of childhood innocence. Indeed, in working with power, mothers can lead and take the discussion about sex forward. Their readiness to do so is pivotal to enabling children's sexual agency to flourish instead of being hidden under the gaze of childhood innocence (Walker 2004). In the context of AIDS, the stakes are high in the continued deployment of childhood innocence and protection as the hegemonic version of childhood. Presuming innocence works to deny the lived experience of many children in this country and diverts attention from the everyday issues that face them.

In this chapter I also explored the social and discursive contexts through which mothers' approaches and practices to AIDS-related knowledge is produced, providing a multifaceted and complex understanding of the social forces through which childhood innocence is upheld and destabilised. AIDS, as many have argued (Patton 1990; Farmer 2006; Fassin 2007; Kippax 2013) is embedded within social, economic, cultural, political and ideological contexts. This is the context through which childhood innocence materialises where power and social inequality are critical.

Discourses of childhood innocence and child protection both shape, and are shaped by, various mothering approaches and experiences. Attention to social context and power remain important. Mothers, as I have argued, do not talk on a blank page. Emerging from opposite ends of the social ladder, the construction of childhood innocence has a historical basis. The current patterns of and reasons for mothers' variations in approaches to and practices in facilitating sexual discussions in AIDS-related knowledge must be understood in interaction with the larger social fabric at KwaDabeka and Bullwood. The social conditions at KwaDabeka that lock in gendered poverty, food scarcity, unemployment, reliance on meagre social grants and male violence to produce dangerous masculinities are the main culprits behind the social construction of child protection. As I have argued in previous chapters, under conditions of ongoing structural inequalities that complexly intertwine with gender inequalities and male vulnerabilities and power to produce violence, children's agency hangs in a noose with girls' particularly squeezed of their power. As Jackson and Scott (2010) argue, the specificities of childhood sexuality are made possible under specific social conditions and frame how they become sexual. At KwaDabeka, mothers, like their children, are rendered vulnerable to, albeit not victims of, material, symbolic and discursive forces which constrain agency and question the very social conditions which allow for the specific construction of sexuality where sexual and gender violence continues to flourish in South Africa, creating vulnerability to HIV (Bhana 2012). The social and cultural dimensions of childhood innocence and child protection are what give it its force and meaning. The discussion with mothers has rendered visible these deeply rooted linkages between childhood innocence, child protection, inequalities, suffering, and power. It also brings attention to abundance and material wealth and prosperity through which stark racial and class inequalities become apparent. As is the case at Bullwood, the context of plenty and historical privilege produces distancing from the contaminating effects of and the racialisation of AIDS—the construction of otherness. AIDS becomes the disease of Africans whilst the children of rich whites remain within the confines of the illusive myth of childhood purity created by separation and wealth. In his wide-ranging and innovative investigations of the nexus of disease and domination, Farmer (2006) has traced how social structures stamped by extreme inequality interact with asymmetric formations of power and knowledge to produce and distribute individual distress and mass illness. Whether at Bullwood or KwaDabeka, the mothers' approaches to children's understanding of AIDS-related knowledge are grounded in a set of practices that contribute further to an environment that is dangerous and antagonistic to children's well-being and safety; reproducing danger, distance and disease as contagion; and invoking asymmetries of power.

Yet as this chapter has shown, AIDS is contradictory, producing childhood innocence and child protection as it opens up the possibility of addressing children's right to and competencies with regard to sexual knowledge. By setting in motion an unusual question to mothers of seven- and eight-year-olds, the interviews have challenged the hegemonic imposition of childhood innocence in the social construction of children's AIDS-related knowledge. AIDS and the question of children's sexual knowledge breaks a silence. At Bullwood, in the context of AIDS amongst whites, Sophie says, "Start looking at yourself . . . what did I do or what didn't I do? I would feel responsible". Questions about facilitating the sexual socialisation of children's AIDS-related knowledge could be a spark that could enhance the mothers' responsibility by examining their assumptions about childhood innocence. As I have demonstrated in this chapter, within the AIDS paradox, the assumed stability of childhood innocence is destabilised and mothers' reflection on their approaches to and practices in relation to the sexual socialisation of children's AIDS-related knowledge is a harbinger of possible change for mediation and appropriate responses.

## REFERENCES

Bernstein, A. (2014) 'South Africa's Key Challenges Tough Choices and New Directions'. *The Annals of the American Academy of Political and Social Science*, 652(1): 20–47.
Bhana, D. (2012) 'Girls Are not Free: In and Out of the South African School'. *International Journal of Educational Development*, 32: 352–358.
Bhana, D. & Nkani, N. (2014) 'When African Teenagers Become Fathers: Culture, Materiality and Masculinity'. *Culture, Health & Sexuality*, 16(4): 337–350.
Bennett, C. & Harden, J. (2014) 'An Exploration of Mothers' Attitudes Towards Their Daughters' Menarche'. *Sex Education: Sexuality, Society and Learning*, 14(4): 457–470.
Butler, J. (2004) *Undoing Gender*. New York: Routledge.
Davies, C. & Robinson, K. (2010) 'Hatching Babies and Stork Deliveries: Risk and Regulation in the Construction of Children's Sexual Knowledge'. *Contemporary Issues in Early Childhood*, 11(3): 249–262.
Egan, R.D. (2013) *Becoming Sexual: A Critical Appraisal of the Sexualization of Girls*. Oxford: Polity Press.
Egan, R.D., & Hawkes, G. (2009) 'The Problem With Protection: Or, Why We Need to Move Towards Recognition and the Sexual Agency of Children'. *Continuum: Journal of Media & Cultural Studies*, 23(3): 389–400.
Epstein, D. & Johnson, R. (1998). *Schooling Sexualities*. Buckingham: Open University Press.
Farmer, P. (2006) *AIDS and Accusation: Haiti and the Geography of Blame*. London: University of California Press.
Fassin, D. (2007). *When Bodies Remember Experiences and Politics of AIDS in South Africa*. Berkeley: University of California Press.

Furedi, F. (2006) *The Politics of Fear; Beyond Left and Right*. London: Continuum Press.

Hunter, M. (2006) 'Fathers Without *Amandla*: Zulu-Speaking Men and Fatherhood', in L. Richter & R. Morrell (eds) *Baba: Men and Fatherhood in South Africa* (pp. 99–107). Pretoria: HSRC.

Hunter, M. (2010) *Love in the Time of AIDS: Inequality, Gender, and Rights in South Africa*. Bloomington: Indiana University Press.

Jackson, S. & Scott, S. (2010) *Theorizing Sexuality*. Maidenhead: McGraw-Hill/Open University Press.

Jewkes, R., Flood, M. & Lang, J. (2014) 'From Work With Men and Boys to Changes of Social Norms and Reduction of Inequities in Gender Relations: A Conceptual Shift in Prevention of Violence Against Women and Girls'. *The Lancet*, 385(9977: 1580-1589): 1–10.

Kaleeba, N. (2004) 'Excerpt From *We Miss You All*: AIDS in the Family', in E. Kalipeni, E. Craddock, S. Oppong & J. Ghosh (eds), *HIV and AIDS in Africa Beyond Epidemiology* (pp. 259–279). Oxford: Blackwell Publishing.

Kawash, S. (2011) 'New Directions in Motherhood Studies'. *Signs*, 36(4): 969–1003.

Kincaid, J. (1998) *Erotic Innocence: The Culture of Child Molesting*. Durham, NC: Duke University Press.

Kitzinger, J. (1998) The gender politics of news production: silenced voices and false memories In C Carter G Branston and S Allan (Eds) News gender power (pp.186-203). London: Routledge.Kippax, S. (2013) 'Effective HIV Prevention: The Indispensable Role of Social Science'. *Journal of the International AIDS Society*, 15(2): 17357.

Martin, K. (2009) 'Normalizing Heterosexuality: Mothers' Assumptions, Talk, and Strategies With Young Children'. *American Sociological Review*, 74: 190–207.

McClintock, A. (1995) *Imperial Leather: Race, Gender and Desire in the Colonial Contest*. New York: Routledge.

O'Reilly, A. (2006) *Rocking the Cradle: Thoughts on Feminism, Motherhood, and the Possibility of Empowered Mothering*. Toronto, ON: Demeter Press.

Pattman, R. (2005) ' "Boys and Girls Should not Be Too Close": Sexuality, the Identities of African Boys and Girls and HIV/AIDS Education'. *Sexualities*, 8(4): 497–516.

Patton, C. (1990) *Inventing AIDS*. New York: Routledge.

Petros, G., Airhihenbuwa, C. O., Simbayi, L., Ramlagan, S. & Brown, B. (2006) 'HIV/AIDS "Othering" in South Africa: The Blame Goes On'. *Culture, Health and Sexuality*, 8(1): 67–77.

Posel, D. (2005) 'Sex, Death and the Fate of the Nation: Reflections on the Politicization of Sexuality in Post-Apartheid South Africa'. *Africa*, 75(2): 125–153.

Renold, E. (2005) *Girls, Boys and Junior Sexualities*. London: RoutledgeFalmer.

Robinson, K. (2013) *Innocence, Knowledge and the Construction of Childhood: The Contradictory Nature of Sexuality and Censorship in Children's Contemporary Lives*. New York: Routledge.

Silin, J. (1995) *Sex, Death and the Education of Children: Our Passion for Ignorance in the Age of AIDS*. New York: Teachers College Press.

Silberschmidt, M. (2001) 'Disempowerment of Men in Rural and Urban East Africa: Implications for Male Identity and Sexual Behavior'. *World Development*, 29(4): 657–671.

Stoller, A. (2002) *Carnal Knowledge and Imperial Power: Race and the Intimate in Colonial Rule*. Berkeley: University of California Press.

Stone, N., Ingham, R. & Gibbins, K. (2013) ' "Where Do Babies Come From?" Barriers to Early Sexuality Communication Between Parents and Young Children'. *Sex Education*, 13(2): 228–240.

Walker, J. (2004) 'Parents and Sex Education: Looking Beyond "the Birds and the Bees" '. *Sex Education*, 4(3): 239–254.

# 8   To Fight Against AIDS, Put Children First

## Rethinking Boys, Girls and Childhood Sexuality

> Children must be at the forefront of the fight against AIDS if countries are to develop, we must put children first.
>
> —UNICEF (2005)

Based on an ethnographic and interview study of children aged between seven and eight (and adult teachers and parents) in two socially diverse South African primary schools, in this book I examined the impact of AIDS in terms of the ways in which gender and sexuality are articulated against the backdrop of race- and class-specific contexts. My approach to this study was that a more capacious view of children that is alert to their agency could provide fresh perspectives on the salience of race, class, gender and sexuality in their meanings of AIDS. I situated children's understanding of AIDS within wider social relations in South Africa, where power, wealth and health are so unevenly distributed. Underwritten by the legacies of apartheid, the social contexts provided rich contextual specificity in children's accounts of the sexual and gendered transmission of the disease. I attended to the varying social means through which children (and adults) interpret, shape and negotiate the sexual and gendered meanings of the disease within the structural parameters of their lives, elucidating the uneven deployment of structural constraints. A central focus in the book has been on the ways in which children actively participate in creating and mediating knowledge of the disease as they transgress, breach, negotiate and promote dominant hegemonic positions of childhood innocence. Throughout the chapters, I have argued that children's understanding of the disease both contests and promotes childhood innocence whilst simultaneously the effect of material, cultural, symbolic and discursive forces creates greater vulnerability for girls. Childhood innocence both constitutes and regulates children's early sexual socialisation (Robinson 2013). Children manoeuvre the social, economic and cultural context of the disease, and their sexual knowledge is embedded within and contingent on these social processes. Of particular significance are the ways in which children's sexual knowledge of the disease provides the leeway to amplify, share and negotiate their complex gendered and sexual selves through various heterosexualising processes including kissing, boyfriends and girlfriends, love letters and marriage, as well as through their discussions of "sleep" (sex) and sexual violence.

In contrast to children's own voices and their sexual, cultural and gendered realities are adult voices (teachers in Chapter 6 and mothers in Chapter 7). Teachers' and mothers' regulation of childhood innocence is critical to the main discussion of AIDS, sex and childhood sexuality. Putting children and sexuality together, as Tobin (1997) suggests, continues to remain problematic and fraught with difficulty. Children do not have access to sexuality and AIDS education and significant adults at home and school do little to address children's sexual knowledge and its relationship to the disease. My interactions with adults about children's knowledge of AIDS broke sexual silences, producing some level of reflection, but adults are largely caught up within notions of childhood innocence and child protection discourses, which regulate and constrain efforts to enhance the sexual health and well-being of children. The nature and form of children's early sexual socialisation from the perspectives of mothers and teachers (at home and at school) reproduces sexual taboos and reinforces childhood purity, innocence and the need for protection. In stark contrast to children's knowledge of the disease, adults relegate and deny access to sexual knowledge in the name of childhood innocence. I have argued that the price of innocence is passivity and continued inattention to children's construction of the disease and to the development of appropriate responses to their needs. Hegemonic versions of childhood innocence are aiding the reproduction of a passive and innocent child. This is troubling from the standpoint of children's right to knowledge and health protection and promotion. Problematic representations about childhood as a time of innocence mean that children's struggles, negotiations and meanings of the disease as they are forged within social circumstances are left uninterrupted, unattended and overlooked. Childhood innocence is discursively constructed. The drivers of children's vulnerability and the focus on the protection of girls from dangerous men and sexual violence, particularly at KwaDabeka, as well as mothers' narratives of their own vulnerability, are rooted within social, economic, cultural and ideological contexts and point to the need to address these fault lines in South African society that continues to create disproportionate vulnerability of African women and girls to HIV whilst leading to a discourse of overprotection and a racialised/classed perception of non-vulnerability at Bullwood. The links between these structural forces and the remnants of apartheid are crucial to understanding gendered and sexual vulnerability and crucial to the understanding of AIDS and what this means in our social responses to it.

In this concluding chapter, I identify some of the key findings from my research with children that expand on the central claims made in this book regarding the ways in which children's AIDS-related sexual knowledge is expressed, negotiated, resisted and regulated. These include the following:

- AIDS is sex: gender and heterosexuality. Children invest in heteronormativity through which gender identities and relations are produced.
- AIDS is sex: gender and sexual danger. Children's knowledge of disease is mediated by gendered vulnerabilities within an overall heteronormative environment calling into question masculinities, violence and the social conditions which produce such violence.
- AIDS stigma: race, gender, class and sexuality. Children's knowledge of disease mediated by race, class and sexual inequalities.
- AIDS, sex and childhood innocence: negotiating age and sexuality.

In contrast, children's AIDS-related sexual knowledge is regulated by adult prescriptions restricting, limiting and reproducing childhood innocence. The chapter then draws from some of the salient points raised by teachers and parents, in Chapters 6 and 7 in rethinking girls', boys' and childhood sexuality. I have identified some of the salient points that deserve attention. Whilst adult teachers and mothers acknowledged the importance of AIDS and sexuality education, childhood sexuality was particularly under siege by adult concerns:

- Age-appropriate knowledge: too young to know
- Silencing sexuality: if children don't ask, don't tell
- Teaching sexuality: teachers fear parents
- Talking about sex initiates sex
- Sexual danger and child protection
- Keep boys and girls apart
- AIDS, the disease of the 'other'

Combined, these findings illustrate how children and adults, located under specific school settings, regulate as they are regulated, by dominant discourses of childhood innocence. These findings illustrate further how far removed adults are from children's social realities. Whilst girls and boys are actively making sense of the disease, expressing both their pleasures and fears as gendered and sexual beings, there is little attention to the development of early sexuality education that is not only important for their health and well-being, especially in the context of AIDS, but also important throughout their lives (Robinson 2013). For too long, too little has been done to reach boys and girls at age seven and eight in addressing AIDS and sexuality education (Bhana *et al.* 2006). In relation to gendering in childhood, Alloway (1995) asserted that "[e]ight's too late". Similarly, as far AIDS, sexuality education and health promotion are concerned, the time is long overdue for a more determined approach that puts children first.

Interventions must begin with children, understanding their agency and vulnerability, where they are and who they are, in order for sexuality education to make sense to them. It would also require bold reflections from adult teachers and parents about what they think children know and what they think children should and should not know in order to fully reflect the complex social processes through which children conceptualise sexual knowledge of disease. For the rest of the chapter, I consider the key findings before turning to the possibility and challenges of working with children in developing AIDS-related sexuality education.

## AIDS IS SEX: GENDER AND HETEROSEXUALITY

### Children Express Sexual Knowledge of the Disease, Debunking Childhood Innocence and Within a Heteronormative Context Through Which Gender Relations and Identities are Produced

Children are social agents. When boys and girls made the connection between AIDS and sex, the opportunity arose to amplify heterosexual desires and investments. In doing so they expressed their agency and debunked the myth of childhood innocence whilst contradictorily inserted within embarrassment, laughter, humour and shame. Children know a great deal about AIDS and although not all know the same things. Knowledge of sex and disease was mixed up with contagion, kissing and dirt and germs. It was through peer support that the myth of childhood innocence was shattered as each child was giving another a point of access to (hetero)sexual (and gendered) cultures. The first point I make here is that children have agency—they are aware, albeit it unevenly, of the sexual transmission of AIDS and they draw from their surrounding social circumstances to express their knowledge of sexuality and disease. Second, whilst they express knowledge of the disease they do so in ways that invoke shame, embarrassment and humour (Allen 2014). Boys and girls are vigilant of their age and role in relation to adults, and specifically their sexual knowledge is often ignored, silenced and underground. Being embarrassed and finding the 'sexual part' of AIDS humorous function to discipline children and to regulate childhood innocence. The embarrassment children feel about sex promotes and validates relations of power and children's place as innocent (Irvine 2002). Indeed, many children distanced from sexual knowledge whilst contradictorily took pleasure in raising the sexual connection of the disease. Distancing from sexuality is an age-appropriate defence strategy to avoid being targeted as non-childlike, contaminated and less than innocent. Children are actively involved in producing, regulating and asserting sexuality whilst promoting childhood innocence. The final point I wish to raise here is that children's investment in sexuality is produced within heteronormative versions of gender. The sexual discussion of the disease produces a complex chain through which heterosexual romance and teasing, kissing (and the links to contagion), sex, condoms, playing tag and boyfriends and girlfriends are explored. When children are given the opportunity and space to talk about AIDS, they connect it with sex and sexuality. In doing so their investments in heterosexuality, desires and pleasures and their gendered narratives are made visible.

## AIDS IS SEX: GENDER AND SEXUAL DANGER

### Children's Knowledge of the Disease Is Mediated by Social Inequalities and an Acute Sense of Girls' Vulnerability to Sexual Violence

Vance (1984) has shown that sexuality is simultaneously a field of restriction, repression and danger, as well as a domain of pleasure and agency, through which gender relations are constructed. On the issue of AIDS, sex and danger, it was clear that girls (and mothers as well) constructed men as dangerous within South Africa's overall climate where sexual and gender violence is rampant (WHO 2013). Children's knowledge of AIDS is strongly influenced by their experiences and their localities. Girls in particular expressed knowledge of disease, danger and vulnerability. At Bullwood and KwaDabeka, the working-class girls made explicit reference to rape and AIDS, with middle-class and working-class girls more generally constructing African men as vectors in the spread of the disease. Children have a sophisticated knowledge of gender inequalities, and a rampant heterosexual masculinity that leads to unsafe and violent sexual relations, which have implications for women and girls. The danger that girls felt at KwaDabeka, as illustrated in Chapter 4, became vividly clear in the discussions of disease, danger and girls' vulnerability leading to the AIDS-is-rape metaphor, where sexuality is framed by and overlaid with fear, which reduces and diminishes agency. As many researchers have suggested children's agency is often restricted and constrained by the social conditions over which they have little control (Parsons 2012; Ansell 2014). Children's responses must be situated within discourses of violent gender and patriarchal relations and their structural location in the township. These ongoing gendered permutations and contestations locate sexuality as a medium through which the disease is represented. Of importance are the ways in which gender relations were produced in the social constitution of sexuality. Boys blamed girls with "G-strings" for driving male sexual violence, producing gendered relations of domination and subordination, while girls blamed boys producing gendered polarities. It was girls in particular, whilst defying the status of helpless victims, who articulated their vulnerability to male violence and rape. Their fear of men is situational, the effect of material, discursive and symbolic forces constraining opportunities and choices available to them. They are certainly at higher risk of rape and disease.

Of special significance here are the real dangers women and girls face where unemployment, poverty and male vulnerabilities coalesce to produce harmful patterns of gender relations and which combined to increase women and girls' vulnerability to danger and disease in township settings. Indeed, a major concern here is not sexuality, but the discourses of childhood innocence, which supposedly protect children from dangerous sexual knowledge.

## AIDS STIGMA: RACE, GENDER, CLASS AND SEXUALITY

### Children's Knowledge of AIDS Is Contradictory, Invokes Care, Contagion and Stigma Which Is Intertwined With Power, Race, Gender, Sexuality and Class Inequalities

AIDS is deeply embedded within gendered, political, ideological and cultural contexts. Chapter 3 argued that children's meanings of the disease weave into the very fabric of power, imbricating wider social relations that both challenge and reproduce inequalities. Throughout the book I have argued that children are social agents as they make meaning of the disease, contesting, challenging and promoting childhood innocence. Pivotal to children's conceptualisations of disease are the social forces through which AIDS-related stigma are produced. At Bullwood, children construct the disease as something to do with Africans, with African men as vectors in the spread of the disease. But they do so in complex ways, mixing contagion with disease and race and with gender, sexuality and class inequalities whilst invoking discourses of care for victims of the disease. First, African men were targeted in the spread of the disease. African men have been particularly problematised in relation to the epidemic, with campaigns addressing them as people with multiple partners perpetrating violence against women and girls (Ratele 2014). Recent campaigns warn young women about dangerous sugar daddies spreading the disease. Children's construction of race and HIV-related stigma takes place in a web of representation of AIDS, which is highly racialised. Second, the economic conditions of the African majority coalesced with contagion and dirt to produce racialised versions of the disease. Children drew on dirt, disease, poverty, sexuality, gender, infection and stigma to construct race and class inequalities. Third, a few children also spoke of the mythical constructs of the disease associating it with witchcraft and sorcery through which conspiracy and racialised views were produced (Nattrass 2006).

Fourth, the complexity of children's meanings to sexuality and disease were illustrated in the contradictory ways in which heterosexuality and gay sex were constructed. Not only do I make claims about children's widespread knowledge of the sexual transmission of the disease. Here I argued also that children's sexuality is caught up in normalised processes of heterosexuality. What was surprising is that whilst the heterosexual spread of the disease has received widespread attention in the country, and from children's own point of view, gay sex, too, was stigmatised. In rejecting gay sexuality, boys and girls were inserting within normative constructions of gender and heterosexuality. Within this complex positioning, children expressed their sexuality whilst also cautioned against it using age categories to distance themselves from sexuality. As the book has argued, knowing too much, too soon can compromise how children are viewed and how they view themselves. Children often positioned themselves as being 'too young to know'. In relation to sexuality, children expressed a great deal of pleasure, but such pleasure, too, was brought under surveillance by childhood innocence. Knowing too much or engaging in sexual activities such as kissing was a complex source of shame and stigma. As other researchers also have argued (Blaise 2005; Renold 2005), sexual ambivalences mark children's experiences of gender and sexuality, and sexual distancing sits alongside sexual pleasures and desires. Finally, locked into the complex power maze of AIDS-stigma were discourses of care. Children spoke about what they would do to support those infected with the disease and were sensitive, empathetic and showed compassion. Instead of a static construction of power/stigma, the findings here complexly intertwine race, class, contagion, sexuality, gender and age showing, too, how care is enmeshed within relations of inequality.

## AIDS, SEX AND CHILDHOOD INNOCENCE: NEGOTIATING AGE AND SEXUALITY

### Children Conceal, Reveal, Negotiate and Hide Sexual Knowledge as Tactical Strategies to Conform and Challenge Childhood Innocence

Children are tactical experts. Their sexual knowledge of AIDS is regulated as they regulate how much they can say, know and express. Chapter 5 considered these contradictions. On one hand, children openly contested childhood innocence by drawing on their sexual knowledge of the disease, but they can also contribute to adults' wish for sexual innocence by distancing from sexuality and drawing on age-appropriate discourses to present the idealisation of innocence. Of importance here is that children are not passive in the construction of childhood innocence; they actively participate in producing adult versions of childhood whilst breaking it down. The resistance to sexual knowledge drew on age-appropriate and developmental discourses. It must be noted here that children's attempts to erase sexuality as inappropriate for age seven and eight stood alongside their pleasures and delight at expressing sexuality—erasure, like pleasure, appeared unpredictably and is part of the complexity as children express, negotiate and hide sexuality. Children's attempts to remove and delay sexual knowledge to a later stage are an attempt by children to adopt adult positions and to project innocence. Children did express concerns about the adult regulatory forces, and this is especially the case at KwaDabeka, where children stated that children who were constructed as naughty and, in this context, as having sexual knowledge would face punitive consequences through corporal punishment. At Bullwood, as I illustrate in Chapter 5, the policing of sexuality is saliently evident when Gugu says, "Don't say anything to the teacher". There were other examples in relation to children's concerns about parents. Whilst children found strategic ways to resist their subordination, their knowledge of sexuality is disciplined by adult authority and power. People with the greatest potential to address sexual matters are least willing to do so. What this means is an uninterrupted mockery of adult insistence of childhood innocence as children subvert, contest and conform to the idealisation of purity. The findings also illustrate that in the absence of sexual knowledge from adults, there are other means including knowledge from peers, access to computers and media.

Children are very skilful—negotiating, resisting and adjusting their right to knowledge of sex and AIDS. The conversations with other boys and girls provided them with opportunities to display or hide their sexuality through a range of contradictory, gendered, 'age-appropriate' discourses. What this suggests is that given the right circumstances, children are very thoughtful and actively negotiate their own sexual predicaments, their pleasures and their concerns. Even at age seven and eight, boys and girls are capable of reflecting on their actual lives and are happy to talk about AIDS and sexuality, but they are also acutely aware of being governed and controlled by discourses of innocence. To act and talk sexually are breaches of order and forms of trouble in themselves and young children know this and are remarkable tactical agents in managing adult concerns and anxieties.

## TOWARDS AN AIDS-FREE GENERATION: CHILDREN FIRST IN SEXUALITY EDUCATION

"Mom, where did I come from?" My mother told me that I fell from heaven. A simple question made my parents uncomfortable; looking for creative ways to avoid answering. Confused, I was reluctant to ask further because I did not want to be disrespectful. Besides, in our community, a child who asks uncomfortable questions can be called all sorts of names like '*nzenza*', a person of loose morals, or '*jeti*', going ahead of her time. I grew up with a strong belief that a good girl should not think about sex, let alone talk about it. This experience is quite common among young girls in Africa as they grow up with so many unanswered questions about their bodies and relationships with boys. Having proper sex education will help girls to answer all these questions. Sex education will help us understand our bodies, sexuality and health needs. It will build our self-confidence and show us how to develop healthy relationships with the opposite sex, avoid unwanted pregnancies and protect ourselves and our future children from HIV. Sex education will tell girls where to go if they need help and how to help others to better understand themselves and build their future. If we want to decrease new HIV infections in Africa, let's start talking about sex and sexuality with our children in our homes, schools and communities.

—UNAIDS (2012: 11)

How do we begin to rethink the tropes that deny childhood sexuality? In South Africa, Life Skills in the Foundation Phase (learners in grades 0–3) as indicated by the Curriculum and Assessment Policy Statement is expected to equip children with knowledge to enhance their personal health and safety and social relationships and to address violence, abuse, AIDS and safety within the broader ambit of rights and respect for others. No mention is made of sexuality in life skills for grades 0 to 3. In South Africa, the National Policy on AIDS for Learners and Educators in Public Schools (Department of Education 1999, 2002) recognises that teachers must provide adequate information and education on AIDS in the context of life skills. Whilst life skills policy does not mention sexuality, this is not an indication of its absence but of its presence in the hidden curriculum (Epstein & Johnson 1998). The children in this study proved themselves to be curious, knowledgeable and capable of thoughtful reflection and their responses, questions and struggles in making sense of the disease is worthy of adult attention. UNESCO (2009) argues for addressing AIDS education, sexuality and gender issues in all stages of schooling. Children as young as five should learn about sexual activity, including kissing, love, caring and physical intimacy as pleasurable aspects of adult lives (see also Bhana *et al.* 2006; Blaise 2009; Robinson 2013). As I have shown in this book, working closely with children, starting where they are at (Renold 2005) and taking their lives and voices seriously have much to offer in rethinking childhood innocence and children's agency. As noted by Save the Children (2007: iii), "[i]n order to make policies and develop programmes which respond to children's needs, parents, teachers, health providers and policy makers have to listen to the views of children. We want to encourage people who work with children to rethink their perceptions and ideas. We are not protecting children by hiding or ignoring facts."

I have shown in this book how adults approach childhood sexuality with trepidation locking into ready-made categories that render children powerless, hiding, ignoring and silencing sexual knowledge of HIV whilst idealising and wishing innocence on children (Epstein & Johnson 1998). Silin (1995: 56) argues that when the topic of the disease is "sanitized, teacher and students are protected from the truly unhealthy aspects of society that might otherwise be revealed; the status quo is ensured". In the rest of this chapter I focus on addressing some of the key issues in working with teachers and parents in disrupting the status quo and addressing sexuality education in children's early lives. A critical component of sexuality education requires attention to children's agency. Boys and girls do not approach the subject of sexuality and disease as blank slates or as innocent. Significantly, it is impossible to frame sexuality education without addressing the heteronormative patterns in children's sexual knowledge and the humour, fun, pleasure, excitement and curiosity through which children approach the sexual component of HIV. It is also important to recognise that whilst boys and girls talk about sex and HIV in engaged ways, they can also hide and conceal their knowledge as they navigate and regulate—and regulate each other—positioning themselves within adult desires for childhood innocence. They are actively making meaning and negotiating their meanings whether adults know this or not and do so in complex ways.

Childhood innocence as a field of power is contradictory, ambivalent, contested and promoted. Boys and girls already have developed an understanding of the sexual connection of the disease although their knowledge is uneven—some know more than others do. As peers they provide the support for knowledge to grow and develop, and in many instances, such knowledge draws from accurate information of sex and sexuality, but this is scattered alongside care and concern, contagion, kissing and damaging racialised/classed and gendered patterns of meaning. In the absence of information and education about sexuality, children are forced to draw on a range of meanings some of which are inaccurate including contagion, evoking the horror of blood and embedded within unequal relations of power. A key argument made in this book is that boys and girls approach the question of HIV, by drawing on their surrounding social circumstances, through which they challenge, contest and negotiate childhood innocence invoking sexuality, gender, race, class and age. Sexuality education might, in itself, not stop girls' particular vulnerability so long as the social conditions in South Africa persist. AIDS, as many have argued, thrives in the fault lines of massive structural inequalities (Schoepf 2004; Farmer 2006; Aggleton et al. 2005) creating a cocktail of toxic patterns of sexual and gender violence and embedded within conditions of poverty and marginalisation. Having noted the limits of sexuality education under circumstances that continue to marginalise children in extreme settings, starting early and addressing children as active agents and building new versions of healthy sexual relationships and gender equality could offer the hope to counter the negative consequences of structural violence (Farmer 2006: xii):

> The more that social inequalities constrain individual agency, the faster HIV spreads . . . AIDS would hasten the death of those unfortunate to

live in poverty and to become infected with HIV and that much could be done to avert the suffering . . .

Sexuality education, however, is not limited to those living in the ebb and flow of violence, poverty and misery. As I have shown, children at Bullwood were already inserting into patterns of thinking and reproducing as they contest, power inequalities, racist stereotypes and Africans, in particular, as vectors in the spread of the disease. The focus on Africans in poverty, as high risk, has, indeed, resulted in a level of reassurance and distancing from the realities of the disease rather than a sense of relevance, and this was evident across the sample of children, teachers and mothers at Bullwood. Children, whether rich or poor, must have the best start in life and access to information that will protect them, if not now then later, from HIV, whilst recognising, too, that it matters very much how information is mediated through social and local circumstances. As UNESCO (2009: 1) notes,

> [e]ffective sexuality education can provide young people with age-appropriate, culturally relevant and scientifically accurate information. It includes structured opportunities for young people to explore their attitudes and values, and to practise the decision-making and other life skills they will need to be able to make informed choices about their sexual lives.

But whilst effective sexuality education remains vital, AIDS is constituted through dynamic interactions and is fully social. Silin (1995: 56), for instance, notes, "just as efforts at prevention cannot be limited to the presentation of risk-reduction strategies, . . . so coming to terms with the social ramifications of AIDS cannot be achieved through a limited focus on scientific knowledge". The social drivers of the AIDS pandemic must be addressed. There are multiple social factors elucidated in this study from the points of view of children, teachers and parents, requiring a multi-pronged response to disease prevention. Alongside a multi-pronged approach to addressing the social aspects of the disease, is an effective sexuality education that recognises ways children's pleasures and pains and relations of power through which meaning of the disease has been constructed. Even at ages seven and eight, boys and girls are capable of reflecting on their actual lives and are happy to talk about AIDS and sexuality. They are aware of its gendered dynamics, but they are also acutely aware of being governed and controlled by discourses of sexual innocence by actively inserting into the hidden and the silence that constitutes much of childhood sexuality.

In rethinking age-appropriate sexual knowledge in AIDS education there is need to challenge existing ideas about children, agency, childhood innocence and sexuality. How do we begin to reconceptualise age-appropriate knowledge when boys and girls already, at ages seven and eight, have sexual knowledge of the disease and actively insert within heteronormative sexual norms? There is urgent need to reframe what is regarded as appropriate.

Robinson (2013), MacNaughton (2000) and Silin (1995) point to several areas of possible disruption including the need for working with parents and building new knowledge about children's sexual agency. Indeed, if sexuality and AIDS education are to be addressed to children, as I have done in this study, then there is a need to address the construction of childhood innocence and its various manifestations:

- Age-appropriate knowledge: too young to know
- Silencing sexuality: if children don't ask, don't tell
- Teaching sexuality: teachers fear parents
- Talking about sex initiates sex
- Sexual danger and child protection
- Keep boys and girls apart
- AIDS, the disease of the 'other'

MacNaughton (2000) argues for a reconceptualisation of the dominant ways in which children are read noting the significance of feminist knowledge. Similarly, there is a need for pre-service and in-service training that takes children, gender and sexuality seriously—a move away from developmental theory to understandings of discourse, power and agency. This will allow for a rethinking of childhood innocence and of the ways in which power, agency and sexuality have effects for teachers, adult parents and children. Beyond this is a need for contextual and social relevance in sexuality and AIDS education. This will require attention to the social and economic context that produces vulnerability and racialised scripts which distance from fuelling racist stereotypes. AIDS implicates all people and the idea that one is safe from the disease based on race and class must be interrogated.

## START WITH CHILDREN

For too long, children younger than ten have been left out of gender, sexuality and health education as agents in their own right. We need start with children, where they are at and put them at the centre of our methodological and theoretical approaches. A fundamental lesson that this book teaches is the obsoleteness of childhood innocence and the mockery of it in light of children's own knowledge of the disease. It also teaches us about the suffering and the effects of large-scale forces on the microcosmic world of children in unequal social contexts as they navigate their little gendered and cultural worlds. As Renold (2005: 178) notes,

> [o]nly by developing a sexuality education which speaks to and connects with children's own gender and sexual cultures can educational

practitioners and policy makers fully support girls' and boys' individual and collective understanding of 'why they feel the ways they do, what it means for the ways they act and what to do about it'.

(Kenway & Fitzclarence, 1997: 30)

It is no easy task to develop a child-centred sexuality and AIDS programmes when children are actively revealing and concealing their sexual knowledge of the disease as they navigate childhood innocence. It is not easy to disrupt ideas of children as innocent when child abuse, and girls particular vulnerability to rape, has taken precedence even in the Sexual Offences Act (2005). However, AIDS does provide a challenge to the continued inattention to the sexual and gendered cultures of children. If we are to address girls' and boys' power and sexualities in dealing with sexuality and AIDS, then we need to seize the opportunity and help address contradictory and constraining discourses of childhood innocence that put the sexual knowledge of AIDS firmly on the agenda. "Children should be the first to benefit from our successes in defeating HIV, and the last to suffer from our failures," observed Anthony Lake, the executive director of UNICEF (2013: 1). The time is long overdue for determined and systematic approach to rethinking children's agency, sexuality and gender and for promoting their sexual health from the very early years of life. I remind the reader of discussion with Cassandra and Natalie about why children should know about AIDS:

Cassandra:   You'll know what AIDS is and you'd know how to get AIDS. You will be more careful.

Natalie:   Because if don't know about it then if you could like get AIDS. You don't know what's wrong with you, you'll think it's a different kind of sickness and you think you're going to die straight away.

Taking on AIDS forcefully would mean a long overdue attention to children not just to hear their voices of the value of AIDS education but also to realise it:

AIDS is above all a remediable adversity. Our living and our life forces are stronger, our capacity for wholeness as humans larger, than the individual effects of the virus. Africa seeks healing. That healing lies within the power of our own actions. In inviting us to deal with the losses it has already inflicted, and, more importantly in enjoining us to avoid future losses that our own capacity to action make necessary, AIDS beckons us to the fullness and power of our own humanity. It is not an invitation that we should avoid or refuse.

(Cameron 2005: 214–215)

## REFERENCES

Aggleton, P., Jenkins, P. & Malcolm, A. (2005) 'HIV/AIDS and Injecting Drug Use: Information, Education and Communication'. *International Journal of Drug Policy*, 16: 21–30.

Allen, L. (2014) 'Don't Forget, Thursday Is Test[icle] Time! The Use of Humour in Sexuality Education', *Sex Education*, 14(4): 387–399.

Alloway, N. (1995) *Foundation Stones: The Construction of Gender in Early Childhood*. Melbourne: Curriculum Corporation.

Ansell, N. (2014) 'Challenging Empowerment: AIDS-Affected Southern African Children and the Need for a Multi-Level Relational Approach'. *Journal of Health Psychology*, 9(1): 22–33.

Bhana, D. & Farook Brixen, F. (with MacNaughton, G. & Zimmerman, R.). (2006) *Young Children, HIV/AIDS and Gender: A Summary Review*. Working paper 39. The Hague, Holland: Bernard van Leer Foundation.

Blaise, M. (2005) 'A Feminist Poststructuralist Study of Children "Doing" Gender in an Urban Kindergarten Classroom'. *Early Childhood Research Quarterly*, 20(1): 85–108.

Blaise, M. (2009) ' "What a Girl Wants, What a Girl Needs": Responding to Sex, Gender, and Sexuality in the Early Childhood Classroom'. *Journal of Research in Childhood Education*, 23(4): 450–460.

Cameron, D. (2005) *Witness to AIDS*. Cape Town: Tafelberg.

Department of Education. (1999) *Revised National Curriculum Statement grade R-9 Life Orientation*. Pretoria: Department of Education.

Epstein, D. & Johnson, R. (1998) *Schooling Sexualities*. Buckingham: Open University Press.

Farmer, P. (2006) *AIDS and Accusation: Haiti and the Geography of Blame*. Berkley: University of California Press.

Irvine, J. M. (2002) *Talk About Sex: The Battles Over Sex Education in the United States*. Berkeley: University of California Press.

Kenway, J. & Fitzclarence, L. (1997) 'Masculinity, Violence and Schooling: Challenging "Poisonous Pedagogies" '. *Gender and Education*, 9(1): 117–134.

MacNaughton, G. (2000) *Rethinking Gender in Early Childhood Education*. London: Paul Chapman.

Nattrass, N. (2006) 'South Africa's "Rollout" of Highly Active Antiretroviral Therapy: A Critical Assessment'. *JAIDS: Journal of Acquired Immune Deficiency Syndromes*, 43(5): 618–623.

Parsons, R. (2012) *Growing Up with HIV in an Eastern Zimbabwean Town. One Day This Will Be Over*. Harare: James Currey, Weaver Press.

Ratele, K. (2014) 'Currents Against Gender Transformation of South African Men: Relocating Marginality to the Centre of Research and Theory of Masculinities'. *NORMA: International Journal for Masculinity Studies*, 9(1): 30–44.

Renold, E. (2005). *Girls, Boys, and Junior Sexualities: Exploring Children's Gender and Sexual Relations in the Primary School*. London: Routledge Falmer.

Robinson, K. (2013) *Innocence, Knowledge and the Construction of Childhood: The Contradictory Nature of Sexuality and Censorship in Children's Contemporary Lives*. New York: Routledge.

Save the Children. (2007) *Tell Me More! Children's Rights and Sexuality in the Context of AIDS in Africa*. Sweden: RFSU.

Schoepf, B. G. (2004) 'AIDS in Africa: Structure, Agency and Risk', in E. Kalipeni, S. Craddock, J. R. Oppong, & J. Ghosh (eds) *AIDS in Africa Beyond Epidemiology* (pp. 121–133). Oxford: Blackwell Publishing.

Silin, J. (1995) *Sex, Death and the Education of Children: Our Passion for Ignorance in the Age of AIDS*. New York: Teachers College Press.

Tobin, J. (1997). 'The Missing Discourse of Pleasure and Desire', in J. Tobin (ed) *Making a Place for Pleasure in Early Childhood Education* (pp. 1–37). New Haven, CT: Yale University Press.

UNAIDS. (2012). *Together We Will End AIDS*. Joint United Nations Program on AIDS: Geneva. UNAIDS.

UNESCO (United Nations Educational, Scientific and Cultural Organization. (2009) *International Technical Guidance on Sexuality Education: An Evidence-informed Approach for Schools*, (Vol. 1 and 2). Paris: Teachers and Health Educators.

UNICEF. (2005) *Unite for Children. Unite Against AIDS A Call to Action: Children, the Missing Face of AIDS*. New York: UNICEF.

UNICEF. (2013) *Towards an AIDS-Free Generation Children and AIDS. Sixth Stocktaking Report*. New York: UNICEF.

Vance, C.S. (ed). (1984) *Pleasure and danger: Exploring Female Sexuality*. New York: Routledge & Kegan Paul Books.

WHO (World Health Organization). (2013) *Global and Regional Estimates of Violence Against Women: Prevalence and Health Effects of Intimate Partner Violence and Non partner Sexual Violence*. Geneva: WHO.

# Bibliography

Aggleton, P. & Campbell, C. (2000) 'Working With Young People—Towards an Agenda for Sexual Health', *Sexual and Relationship Therapy*, 15(3): 283–296.

Aggleton, P., Jenkins, P. & Malcolm, A. (2005) 'HIV/AIDS and Injecting Drug Use: Information, Education and Communication'. *International Journal of Drug Policy*, 16: 21–30.

Aggleton, P., Yankah, E. & Crewe, M. (2011) 'Education and HIV/AIDS— 30 Years on'. *AIDS Education and Prevention*, 23(6): 495–507.

Alanen, L. (1997) 'The Politics of Growing Up'. Paper presented at a seminar at Keele University, March.

Alderson, P. (2007)' Competent Children? Minors' Consent to Health Care Treatment and Research'. *Social Science and Medicine*, 65: 2272–2283.

Allen, L. (2011) *Young People and Sexuality Education: Rethinking Key Debates.* New York: Palgrave Macmillan.

Allen, L. (2014) 'Don't Forget, Thursday Is Test[icle] Time! The Use of Humour in Sexuality Education', *Sex Education*, 14(4): 387–399.

Alloway, N. (1995) *Foundation Stones: The Construction of Gender in Early Childhood*. Melbourne: Curriculum Corporation.

Ansell, N. (2014) 'Challenging Empowerment: AIDS-Affected Southern African Children and the Need for a Multi-Level Relational Approach'. *Journal of Health Psychology*, 9(1): 22–33.

Banas, J., Dunbar, N., Rodriguez, D. & Liu. S. (2011) 'A Review of Humor in Educational Settings: Four Decades of Research'. *Communication Education*, 60(1): 115–144.

Barbarin, O. A. & Richter, L. (2001) *Mandela's Children*. New York: Routledge.

Barnes, C. (2012) 'It's No Laughing Matter . . . Boys' Humour and the Performance of Defensive Masculinities in the Classroom'. *Journal of Gender Studies*, 21(3): 239–251.

Baxen, J. and Breidlid, A. (Eds.) (2009). HIV/AIDS in Sub-Saharan Africa. Understanding the Implications of Culture and Context. Cape Town: UCT Press.

Bennett, C. & Harden, J. (2014) 'An Exploration of Mothers' Attitudes Towards Their Daughters' Menarche'. *Sex Education: Sexuality, Society and Learning*, 14(4): 457–470.

Bernstein, A. (2014) 'South Africa's Key Challenges Tough Choices and New Directions'. *The Annals of the American Academy of Political and Social Science*, 652(1): 20–47.

Bhana, D. (2006) 'The (Im)Possibility of Child Sexual Rights in Young South African Children's Account of HIV/AIDS'. *IDS Bulletin*, 37(4): 64–68.

Bhana, D. (2007) 'The Price of Innocence: Teachers, Gender, Childhood Sexuality, HIV and AIDS in Early Schooling'. *International Journal of Inclusive Education*, 11(4): 431–444.

Bhana, D. (2007) 'Childhood Sexualities and Rights in HIV contexts'. *Culture Health & Sexuality*, 9(3): 309–324.

Bhana, D. (2008) 'Beyond Stigma? Young Children's Responses to HIV and AIDS'. *Culture, Health & Sexuality*, 10(7): 725–738.

Bhana, D. (2008) '"Six Packs and Big Muscles, and Stuff Like That" Primary School-Aged South African Boys Black and White, on Sport'. *British Journal of Sociology of Education*, 29(1): 3–14.

Bhana, D. (2012) '"Girls Are not Free" in and out of the South African School'. *International Journal of Educational Development*, 32(2): 352–358.

Bhana, D. (2013) 'Kiss and Tell: Boys, Girls and Sexualities in the Early Years'. *Agenda*, 27(3): 57–66.

Bhana, D. & Farook Brixen, F. (with MacNaughton, G. & Zimmerman, R.). (2006) *Young Children, HIV/AIDS and Gender: A Summary Review*. Working paper 39. The Hague: Bernard van Leer Foundation.

Bhana, D. & Nkani, N. (2014) 'When African Teenagers Become Fathers: Culture, Materiality and Masculinity'. *Culture, Health & Sexuality*, 16(4): 337–350.

Bhana, D. & Singh, S. (2012) 'Gender, Sexuality and HIV and AIDS Education in South Africa'. *The Impact of HIV/AIDS on Education Worldwide*, 18: 213–230.

Bhana, D. & Epstein, D. (2007) ' "I Don't Want to Catch It" Boys, Girls and Sexualities in an HIV Environment'. *Gender and Education*, 19(1): 109–125.

Blaise, M. (2005) *Playing it Straight: Uncovering Gender Discourses in the Early Childhood Classroom*. London & New York: Routledge.

Blaise, M. (2005) 'A Feminist Poststructuralist Study of Children "Doing" Gender in an Urban Kindergarten Classroom'. *Early Childhood Research Quarterly*, 20(1): 85–108.

Blaise, M. (2009) ' "What a Girl Wants, What a Girl Needs": Responding to Sex, Gender, and Sexuality in the Early Childhood Classroom'. *Journal of Research in Childhood Education*, 23(4): 450–460.

Blaise, M. (2010) 'Kiss and Tell: Gendered Narratives in Childhood Sexuality'. *Australasian Journal of Early Childhood*, 35(1): 1–9.

Boyce, P., Huang Soo Lee, M., Jenkins, C., Mohamed, S., Overs, C., Paiva, V. & Aggleton, P. (2007) 'Putting Sexuality (Back) into HIV/AIDS: Issues, Theory and Practice 1'. *Global Public Health*, 2(1): 1–34.

Bray, R., Gooskens, I., Kahn, L., Moses, S. & Seekings, J. (2010) *Growing Up in the New South Africa: Childhood and Adolescence in the New South Africa*. Cape Town: Human Sciences, Research Council Press.

Brown, L. Macintyre, K. & Trujillo, T. (2003) 'Interventions to Reduce HIV-Related Stigma: What Have We Learned'. *AIDS Education & Prevention*, 15: 49–69.

Burman, S.B. & Reynolds, P. (eds). (1986) *Growing Up in a Divided Society: The Contexts of Childhood in South Africa*. Johannesburg: Raven Press.

Butler, J. (1990) *Gender Trouble: Feminism and the Subversion of Identity*. New York: Routledge.

Butler, J. (2004) *Undoing Gender*. New York: Routledge.

Cameron, D. (2005). *Witness to AIDS*. Cape Town: Tafelberg.

Campbell, C. (2003) *Letting Them Die: Why HIV/AIDS Intervention Programmes Fail*. Oxford: James Curry.

Campbell, C., Foullis, CA. Maimane, S. & Sibiya, Z. (2005) ' "I Have an Evil Child at My House". Stigma and HIV/AIDS Management in a South African Community'. *American Journal of Public Health*, 95: 808–815.

Campbell, C., Nair, Y., Maimane, S. & Nicholson, J. (2007) 'A Multi-Level Model of Roots in HIV-Related Stigma in Two South African Communities'. *Journal of Health Psychology*, 12(3): 403–416.

Carton, B. (2001) 'Locusts Fall from the Sky: Manhood and Migrancy in KwaZulu', in R. Morrell (ed) *Changing Men in South Africa* (pp. 129–140). Pietermaritzburg: University of Natal Press.

Castro, A. & Farmer, P. (2005) 'Understanding and Addressing HIV-Related Stigma: From Anthropological Theory to Clinical Practice in Haiti'. *American Journal of Public Health*, 95(1): 53–59.

Chase, E. & Aggleton, P. (2006) 'Meeting the Sexual Health Needs of Young People Living on the Street', in R. Ingham & P. Aggleton (eds) *Promoting Young People's Sexual Health* (pp. 81–98). London: Routledge.

Chong, E., Hallman, K. & Brady, M. (2006). *Investing When it Counts*. New York: UNFPA and Population Council.

Clark, J. (2014) 'Sexualisation and the Discursive Figure of the Child', *Sociological Studies of Children and Youth*, 18: 173–197.

Cobbett, M., McLaughlin, C. & Kiragu, S. (2013) 'Creating "Participatory Spaces": Involving Children in Planning Sex Education Lessons in Kenya, Ghana and Swaziland'. *Sex Education*, 13(1): 70–83.

Corrêa, S., Petchesky, R. & Parker, R. (2008) *Sexuality, Health and Human Rights*. London: Routledge.

Craddock, S. (2004) 'Beyond Epidemiology: Locating AIDS in Africa', in E. Kalipeni, E. Craddock, S. Oppong & J. Ghosh (eds) *AIDS in Africa Beyond Epidemiology* (pp. 1–10). Oxford: Blackwell Publishing.

Davies, B. (1993) *Shards of Glass: Children Reading and Writing Beyond Gendered Identities*. St. Leonards, NSW: Allen and Unwin.

Davies, C. & Robinson, K. (2010) 'Hatching Babies and Stork Deliveries: Risk and Regulation in the Construction of Children's Sexual Knowledge'. *Contemporary Issues in Early Childhood*, 11(3): 249–262.

Delius, P. & Glaser, C. (2002). 'Sexual Socialization in South Africa: A Historical Perspective'. *African Studies*, 61: 27–54.

Delius, P. & Glaser, C. (2005) 'Sex, Disease and Stigma in South Africa: Historical Perspectives'. *African Journal of AIDS Research*, 4(1): 29–36.

Department of Education. (1996). *South African Schools Act*. Department of Education, Pretoria, South Africa.

Department of Education. (1998) *National Norms and Standards*. Pretoria: Department of Education.

Department of Education. (1999) *Revised National Curriculum Statement grade R-9 Life Orientation*. Pretoria: Department of Education.

Department of Education. (2006) *Amended National Norms and Standards for School Funding*. Pretoria: Department of Education.

Department of Health. (2005) *Summary Report: National HIV and Syphilis Antenatal Sero-Prevalence Survey in South Africa 2002*. Department of Health, Health Systems Research, Research Coordination and Epidemiology, Republic of South Africa.

Egan, R.D. (2013) *Becoming Sexual: A Critical Appraisal of the Sexualization of Girls*. Oxford: Polity Press.

Egan, R.D. & Hawkes, G. (2009) 'The Problem With Protection: Or, Why We Need to Move Towards Recognition and the Sexual Agency of Children'. *Continuum: Journal of Media & Cultural Studies*, 23(3): 389–400.

Epstein, D. & Johnson, R. (1998) *Schooling Sexualities*. Buckingham: Open University Press.

Epstein, D., O'Flynn, S. & Telford, D. (2003) *Silenced Sexualities in Schools and Universities*. Stoke-on-Trent: Trentham Books.

Farmer, P. (2004) 'An Anthropology of Structural Violence 1'. *Current anthropology*, 45(3): 305–325.

Farmer, P. (2006) *AIDS and Accusation: Haiti and the Geography of Blame*. London: University of California Press.

Fassin, D. (2007). *When Bodies Remember: Experiences and Politics of AIDS in South Africa*. London: University of California Press.

Foucault, M. (1977) *Discipline and Punish*: New York: Pantheon.

Foucault, M. (1978) *The Will to Knowledge: The History of sexuality, volume 1* (Trans. R. Hurley). Harmondsworth: Penguin.

Foucault, M. (1980) *Power/Knowledge: Selected Interviews and Other Writings 1972–1977*. Hemel Hempstead: Harvester.

Francis, D. A. (2012) 'Teacher Positioning on the Teaching of Sexual Diversity in South African Schools'. *Culture, Health & Sexuality*, 14(6): 69–76.

Frosh, S., Phoenix, A. & Pattman, R. (2002) *Young Masculinities: Understanding Boys in Contemporary Society*. London: Palgrave.

Furedi, F. (2006) *The Politics of Fear: Beyond Left and Right*. London: Continuum Press.

Fuss, D. (1989) *Essentially Speaking: Feminism, Nature and Difference*. New York: Routledge.

Galtung, J. (1969) 'Violence, Peace and Peace Research'. *Journal of Peace Research*, 6: 167–191.

Goffman, E. (1963) *Stigma: Notes on the Management of Spoiled Identity*. Englewood Cliffs, NJ: Prentice Hall.

Hallman, K. (2007) 'Sexuality, Reproductive Health and HIV/AIDS: Non-Consensual Sex, School Enrolment and Educational Outcomes in South Africa'. *Africa Insight*, 37(3): 454–472.

Harrison, A. (2008) 'Hidden Love: Sexual Ideologies and Relationship Ideals Among Rural South African Adolescents in the Context of HIV/AIDS'. *Culture Health and Sexuality*, 10(2): 175–189.

Heinze, E. (ed). (2000) *Of Innocence and Autonomy Children, Sex and Human Rights*. Aldershot: Ashgate.

Henderson, P. C. (2006) 'South African AIDS Orphans: Examining Assumptions Around Vulnerability From the Perspective of Rural Children and Youth'. *Childhood*, 13(3): 303–327.

Hey, V. (1997) *The Company She Keeps: An Ethnography of Girls' Friendships*. Buckingham: Open University Press.

Holland, P. (2004) *Picturing Childhood: The Myth of the Child in Popular Imagery*. London: I. B. Tauris.

Human Rights Watch. (2001) *Scared at School: Sexual Violence Against Girls in South African Schools*. Washington DC: Human Rights Watch.

Human Rights Watch. (2001) *Scared at school: sexual violence against girls in South African schools*. New York: Human Rights Watch.

HSRC (Human Sciences Research Council). (2002) *Nelson Mandela HSRC study of AIDS*. Cape Town: HSRC Press.

HSRC (Human Sciences Research Council). (2005) *South African National HIV Prevalence, HIV Incidence, Behaviour and Communication Survey, 2005*. Cape Town: HSRC Press.

Hunter, M. (2005) 'Cultural Politics and Masculinities: Multiple-Partners in Historical Perspective in KwaZulu-Natal'. *Culture, Health and Sexuality*, 7: 389–403.

Hunter, M. (2006) 'Fathers Without *Amandla*: Zulu-Speaking Men and Fatherhood', in L. Richter & R. Morrell (eds) *Baba: Men and Fatherhood in South Africa* (pp. 99–107). Pretoria: HSRC.

Hunter, M. (2007) 'The Changing Political Economy of Sex in South Africa: The Significance of Unemployment and Inequalities to the Scale of the AIDS Pandemic'. *Social Science & Medicine*, 64(3): 689–700.

Hunter, M. (2010) *Love in the Time of AIDS: Inequality, Gender, and Rights in South Africa*. Bloomington: Indiana University Press.

Ingraham, C. (1996) 'The Heterosexual Imaginary: Feminist Sociology and Theories of Gender', in S. Seidman (ed) *Queer Theory/Sociology* (pp. 168–193). Cambridge, MA: Blackwell.

Irvine, J. M. (2002) *Talk About Sex: The Battles Over Sex Education in the United States*. Berkeley: University of California Press.

Iyer, P. & Aggleton, P. (2012) ' "Sexuality Education Should Be Taught, Fine . . . But We Make Sure They Control Themselves": Teachers' Beliefs and Attitudes Towards Young People's Sexual and Reproductive Health in a Ugandan Secondary School.' *Sex Education*, 13(1): 40–53.

Jackson, S. & Scott, S. (2010) *Theorizing Sexuality*. Maidenhead: McGraw-Hill/Open University Press.

James, A., Jenks, C. & Prout, A. (1998) *Theorising Childhood*. Cambridge: Polity Press.

Janssen, D. F. (2002) *Growing Up Sexually (Interim Report), October 2002. Volume 2: The Sexual Curriculum: The Manufacture and Performance of Pre-Adult Sexualities*. Amsterdam. Available online: http://www2.hu-berlin.de/sexology/GESUND/ARCHIV/GUS/INDEX.HTM.

Jewkes, R. (2006) Beyond Stigma: Social Responses to HIV in South Africa. *The Lancet*, 368(9534): 430–431.

Jewkes, R. & Abrahams, N. (2002) 'The Epidemiology of Rape and Sexual Coercion in South Africa: An Overview'. *Social Science and Medicine*, 55: 1231–1244.

Jewkes, R. & Morrell, R. (2012) 'Sexuality and the Limits of Agency Among South African Teenage Women: Theorising Femininities and Their Connections to HIV Risk Practises'. *Social Science & Medicine*, 74(11): 1729–1737.

Jewkes, R., Dunkle, K., Koss, M. P., Levin, J. B., Ndunae, M., Jamaa, N. & Sikweyiya, Y. (2006) 'Rape Perpetration by Young, Rural South African Men: Prevalence, Patterns and Risk Factors'. *Social Science & Medicine*, 63: 2949–2961.

Jewkes, R., Flood, M. & Lang, J. (2014) 'From Work With Men and Boys to Changes of Social Norms and Reduction of Inequities in Gender Relations: A Conceptual Shift in Prevention of Violence Against Women and Girls'. *The Lancet*, 395 (9977): 1580–1589.

Jewkes, R., Levin, J., Mbananga, N. & Bradshaw, D. (2002) 'Rape of Girls in South Africa'. *Lancet*, 359: 319–320.

Jewkes, R., Penn-Kekana, L. & Rose-Junius, H. (2005) ' "If They Rape Me, I Can't Blame Them": Reflections on Gender in the Social Context of Child Rape in South Africa and Namibia'. *Social Science & Medicine*, 61: 1809–1820

Johnson, R. L., Sendall, M. C. & McCuaig, L. A. (2014) 'Primary Schools and the Delivery of Relationships and Sexuality Education: The Experience of Queensland Teachers'. *Sex Education: Sexuality, Society and Learning*, 14(4): 359–374.

Jones, S. (1993) *Assaulting Childhood: Children's Experiences of Migrancy and Hostel Life in South Africa*. Johannesburg: Witwatersrand University Press.

Kaleeba, N. (2004) 'Excerpt From *We Miss You All*: AIDS in the Family', in E. Kalipeni, E. Craddock, S. Oppong & J. Ghosh (eds) *HIV and AIDS in Africa Beyond Epidemiology* (pp. 259–279). Oxford: Blackwell Publishing.

Kalichman, S. C., Simbayi, L. C., Jooste, S., Toefy, Y., Cain, D., Cherry, C. & Kagee, A. (2005) 'Development of a Brief Scale to Measure AIDS-Related Stigma in South Africa'. *AIDS Behaviour*, 9: 35–143.

Kane, E. W. (2013) *Rethinking Gender and Sexuality in Childhood*. New York: Bloomsbury.

Karim, Q. A., Kharsany, A.B.M., Leask, K., Ntombela, F., Humphries, H., Frohlich, J. A., Samsunder, N., Grobler, A., Dellar, R. & Karim, S.S.A. (2014) 'Prevalence of HIV, HSV-2 and Pregnancy Among High School Students in Rural KwaZulu-Natal, South Africa: A Bio-Behavioural Cross-Sectional Survey'. *Epidemiology*, 90(8): 620–627.

Kawash, S. (2011) 'New Directions in Motherhood Studies'. *Signs*, 36(4): 969–1003.

Kehily, M. (ed). (2004) *An Introduction to Childhood Studies*. Buckingham: Open University Press/McGraw Hill.

Kehily, M. & Nayak, A. (1997) 'Lads and Laughter: Humour and the Production of Heterosexual Hierarchies'. *Gender and Education*, 9 (1): 69–87.

Kenway, J. & Fitzclarence, L. (1997) 'Masculinity, Violence and Schooling: Challenging "Poisonous Pedagogies"'. *Gender and Education*, 9(1): 117–134.

Kincaid, J. (1994) *Child Loving: The Erotic Child and Victorian Culture*. New York: Routledge.

Kincaid, J.R. (1998) *Erotic Innocence: The Culture of Child Molesting*. Durham, NC: Duke University Press.

Kippax, S. (2013) 'Effective HIV Prevention: The Indispensable Role of Social Science'. *Journal of the International AIDS Society*, 15(2): 17357.

Kippax, S., Stephenson, N., Parker, R.G. & Aggleton, P. (2013) 'Between Individual Agency and Structure in HIV Prevention: Understanding the Middle Ground of Social Practice'. *American Journal of Public Health*, 103(8): 1367–1375.

Kitzinger, J. (1998) The gender politics of news production: silenced voices and false memories In C Carter G Branston and S Allan (Eds) *News gender power* (pp.186-203). London: Routledge.Le Clerc Madlala, S. (2001). 'Virginity Testing: Managing Sexuality in a Maturing HIV/AIDS Epidemic'. *Medical Anthropology Quarterly*, 15(4): 533–553.

MacNaughton, G. (2000) *Rethinking Gender in Early Childhood Education*. London: Paul Chapman Publishing.

Mager, A. (1999). *Gender and the Making of a South African Bantustan: A Social History of the Ciskei 1945–1959*. Portsmouth, NH: Heinemann.

Magni, S. & Reddy, V. (2007). 'Performative Queer Identities: Masculinities and Public Bathroom Usage'. *Sexualities*, 10(2): 229–242.

*Mail & Guardian* (19 February 2008). 'Outrage Over Attack on Mini Skirt-Wearing Woman'. http://www.mg.co.za/article/2008–02–19-outrage-over-attack-on-miniskirtwearing-woman, accessed 10 July 2008.

Mane, P. & Aggleton, P. (2001). 'Gender and HIV/AIDS: What Do Men Have to Do With it?' *Current Sociology*, 49: 23–38.

Martin, K. (2009) 'Normalizing Heterosexuality: Mothers' Assumptions, Talk, and Strategies With Young Children'. *American Sociological Review*, 74: 190–207.

Mayall, B. (2002) *Towards a Sociology of Childhood: Thinking from Children's Lives*. Buckingham: Open University Press.

Maylam, P. & Edwards, L. (eds). (1995) *The People's City African Life in Twentieth-Century* Durban: University of Natal Press.

McClendon, T. (2006) 'You Are What You Eat Up: Deposing Chiefs in Early Colonial Natal, 1847–58'. *The Journal of African History*, 47: 259–279.

McClintock, A. (1995) *Imperial Leather: Race, Gender and Sexuality in the Colonial Conquest*. London: Routledge.

Measor, L., Tiffin, C. & Fry, K. (1996) 'Gender and Sex Education: A Study of Adolescent Responses'. *Gender and Education*, 8 (3): 275–288.

Mellor, J.D. & Epstein, D. (2006) 'Sexualities and Schooling', in C. Skelton, B. Francis & L. Smulyan (eds) *Handbook of Gender and Education* (pp. 378–391). Thousand Oaks, CA: Sage.

Miedema, E., Maxwell, C. & Aggleton, P. (2015) 'The Unfinished Nature of Rights Informed HIV- and AIDS-Related Education: An Analysis of Three School-Based Initiatives'. *Sex Education: Sexuality, Society and Learning*, 15(1): 78–92.

Moffett, H. (2006). ' "These Women, They Force Us to Rape Them": Rape as Narrative of Social Control in Post-Apartheid South Africa'. *Journal of Southern African Studies*, 32(1): 131–144.

Morrell, R., Epstein, D., Unterhalter, E., Bhana, D. & Moletsane, R. (2009) *Towards Gender Equality? South African Schools During the HIV/AIDS Epidemic*. Pietermaritzburg: University of KwaZulu-Natal Press.

Namisi, F. S., Flisher, A. J., Overland, S., Bastien, S., Onya, H., Kaaya, S. & Aarø, L. E. (2009) 'Socio-Demographic Variations in Communication on Sexuality and HIV/ AIDS With Parents, Family Members and Teachers among in School-Adolescents: A Multi-Site Study in Tanzania and South Africa'. *Scandinavian Journal of Public Health*, 37: 65–74.

Nattrass, N. (2004) *The Moral Economy of AIDS in South Africa*. Cambridge: Cambridge University Press.

Nattrass, N. (2006) 'South Africa's "Rollout" of Highly Active Antiretroviral Therapy: A Critical Assessment'. *JAIDS: Journal of Acquired Immune Deficiency Syndromes*, 43(5): 618–623.

Natrass, N. (2013) 'Understanding the Origins and Prevalence of AIDS Conspiracy Beliefs in the United States and South Africa', *Sociology of Health and Illness*,35(1):113-29.Nayak, A. & Kehily, M. J. (2001). '"Learning to Laugh": A Study of Schoolboy Humour in the English Secondary School', in W. Martino & B. Meyenn (eds) *What About The Boys? Issues of Masculinity in Schools* (pp. 110–124). Buckingham: Open University Press.

Norman, A., Chopra, M. A. & Kadiyala, S. (2007) 'Factors Related to HIV Disclosure in 2 South African Communities'. *American Journal of Public Health*, 97(10): 1775–1781.

O'Reilly, A. (2006) *Rocking the Cradle: Thoughts on Feminism, Motherhood, and the Possibility of Empowered Mothering*. Toronto, ON: Demeter Press.

Parker, R. (2009) 'Sexuality, Culture and Society: Shifting Paradigms in Sexuality Research'. *Culture, Health & Sexuality: An International Journal for Research, Intervention and Care*, 11(3): 251–266.

Parker, R. (2010) 'Reinventing Sexual Scripts: Sexuality and Social Change in the Twenty-First Century'. *Sexuality Research and Social Policy*, 7(1): 58–66.

Parker, R. & Aggleton, P. (2003) 'HIV and AIDS-Related Stigma and Discrimination: A Conceptual Framework and Implications for Action'. *Social Science & Medicine*, 57(1): 13–24.

Parkes, J. (2008). 'The Multiple Meanings of Violence. Children's Talk About Life in a South African Neighbourhood'. *Childhood*, 14(4): 401–414.

Parsons, R. (2012) *Growing Up With HIV in Zimbabwe. One Day This Will Be Over*. Harare: James Currey, Weaver Press.

Pattman, R. (2005) '"Boys and Girls Should not Get Too Close": Sexuality, the Identities of African Boys and Girls and HIV/AIDS Education'. *Sexualities*, 8(4): 501–520.

Pattman, R. & Bhana, D. (2006) 'Black Boys With Bad Reputations'. *Alternations*, 13(2): 252–272.

Pattman, R. & Chege, F. (2003) *Finding Our Voices: Gendered and Sexual Identities in HIV/AIDS Education*. Nairobi: UNICEF ESARO.

Patton, C. (1990) *Inventing AIDS*. New York: Routledge.

Patton, C. (1996) *Fatal Advice: How Safe-Sexuality Education Went Wrong*. Durham, NC: Duke University Press.

Pendry, B. (1998) 'The Links Between Gender Violence and HIV/AIDS'. *Agenda*, 39: 30–33.

Petros, G., Airhihenbuwa, H., Simbayi, L., Ramlagan, S. & Brown, B. (2006) 'HIV/ AIDS and 'Othering' in South Africa: The Blame Goes On'. *Culture, Health and Sexuality*, 8(1): 67–77.

Pettifor, A. E., Rees, H. V., Steffenson, A., Hlongwa-Madikizela, L., Macphail, C., Vermaak, K. & Kleinschmidt, I. (2004). *HIV and Sexual Behaviour Among Young South Africans: National Survey of 15–24 year-olds*. Reproductive Health Research Unit, University of Witwatersrand, Johannesburg.

Posel, D. (2005) 'Sex, Death and the Fate of the Nation: Reflections on the Politicization of Sexuality in Post-Apartheid South Africa'. *Africa*, 75(2): 125–153.

Posel, D. (2005) 'The Scandal of Manhood: "Baby Rape" and the Politicization of Sexual Violence in Post-Apartheid South Africa'. *Culture Health and Sexuality*, 7(3): 239–252.

Pred, A. (2000) *Even in Sweden: Racisms, Racialised Spaces and the Popular Geographical Imagination*. Berkeley: University of California Press.

Pulerwitz, J. & Bongaarts, J. (2014) 'Tackling Stigma: Fundamental to an AIDS-Free Future'. *The Lancet Global Health*, 2(6): e311–e312.

Ramphele, M. (2002) *Steering by the Stars: Being Young in South Africa*. Cape Town: Tafelberg.

Ratele, K. (2014) 'Currents Against Gender Transformation of South African Men: Relocating Marginality to the Centre of Research and Theory of Masculinities'. *NORMA: International Journal for Masculinity Studies*, 9(1): 30–44.

Reddy, V. (2004) 'Sexuality in Africa: Some Trends, Transgressions and Tirades'. *Agenda*, 62: 3–11.

Renold, E. (2005) *Girls, Boys, and Junior Sexualities: Exploring Children's Gender and Sexual Relations in the Primary School*. London: RoutledgeFalmer.

Reynolds, P. (1989) *Childhood in Crossroads: Cognition and society in South Africa*. Cape Town: David Phillip Grand Rapids.

Richter, L. (2004) 'The Impact of HIV/AIDS on the Development of Children', in P. Robyn (ed) *A Generation at Risk HIV/AIDS Vulnerable Children and Security in Southern Africa* (pp. 9–33). Pretoria: Institute for Security Studies.

Richter, L.M., Dawes, A. & Higson-Smith, C. (eds). (2004) *Sexual Abuse of Young Children in Southern Africa*. Pretoria: HSRC Press.

Robinson, K. (2013) *Innocence, Knowledge and the Construction of Childhood: The Contradictory Nature of Sexuality and Censorship in Children's Contemporary lives*. New York: Routledge.

Robinson, K.H. (2005) 'Childhood and Sexuality: Adult Constructions and Silenced Children', in J. Mason & T. Fattore (eds) *Children Taken Seriously in Theory, Policy and Practice* (pp. 66–78). London: Jessica Kingsley.

Robinson, S. (2013) 'Regulating the Race: Aboriginal Children in Private European Homes in Colonial Australia'. *Journal of Australian Studies*, 37(3): 302–315.

Save the Children. (2007) *Tell Me More! Children's Rights and Sexuality in the Context of AIDS in Africa*. Stockholm: RFSU.

Schoepf, B. G. (2004). 'AIDS in Africa: Structure, Agency and Risk', in E. Kalipeni, E. Craddock, S. Oppong & J. Ghosh (eds) *AIDS in Africa Beyond Epidemiology* (pp. 121–133). Oxford: Blackwell Publishing.

Sears, J. (ed). (1992) *Sexuality and the Curriculum*. New York: Teachers College Press.

Sedgwick, E.K. (1990) *The Epistemology of the Closet*. Berkeley: University of California Press.

Shisana, O. & Simbayi, L. (2002) *South African National HIV Prevalence, Behavioural Risks and Mass Media Household Survey*. Cape Town: HSRC Publishers.

Shisana, O., Rehle, T. & Simbayi, L.C. (2005) *South African National HIV Prevalence, HIV Incidence, Behaviour and Communication Survey*. Cape Town: Human Sciences Research Council.

Shisana, O., Rehle, T., Simbayi, L.C., Zuma, K., Jooste, S. & Zungu, N. (2014) South African National HIV Prevalence, Incidence and Behaviour Survey, 2012. Cape Town: HSRC Press.

Silberschmidt, M. (2001) 'Disempowerment of Men in Rural and Urban East Africa: Implications for Male Identity and Sexual Behavior'. *World Development*, 29(4): 657–671.

Silin, J. (1995) *Sex, Death and the Education of Children: Our Passion for Ignorance in the Age of AIDS*. New York: Teachers College Press.

Statistics South Africa. (2014) *Mid-Year Population Estimates*. Pretoria: Statistics South Africa.

Stoller, A. (2002) *Carnal Knowledge and Imperial Power: Race and the Intimate in Colonial Rule*. Berkeley: University of California Press.

Stone, N., Ingham, R. & Gibbins, K. (2013) ' "Where Do Babies Come From?" Barriers to Early Sexuality Communication Between Parents and Young Children'. *Sex Education*, 13(2): 228–240.

Taylor, Y. (ed). (2010) *Classed Intersections: Space, Selves, Knowledges*. Aldershot: Ashgate.

Thamm, M. (2002) *I Have Life: Alison's Journey as Told to Marianne Thamm*. Johannesburg: The Penguin Group.

Therborn, G. (2013) *The Killing Fields of Inequality*. Cambridge: Polity Press.

Thorne, B. (1993). *Gender Play: Girls and Boys in School*. New Brunswick, NJ: Rutgers University Press.

Tobin, J. (ed). (1997) *Making a Place for Pleasure in Early Childhood Education*. New Haven, CT: Yale University Press.

Treichler, P. A. (1999) *How to Have Theory in an Epidemic: Cultural Chronicles of AIDS*. Durham, NC: Duke University Press.

UNAIDS. (2004) *Executive Summary: 2004 Report on the Global AIDS Epidemic*. New York: UNAIDS.

UNAIDS. (2012). *Together We Will End AIDS*. Joint United Nations Program on AIDS. Geneva: UNAIDS.

UNESCO (United Nations Educational, Scientific and Cultural Organization). (2009) *International Technical Guidance on Sexuality Education: An Evidence-Informed Approach for Schools, Teachers and Health Educators, Vol 1—Rationale for Sexuality Education*. Paris: UNESCO.

UNESCO (United Nations Educational, Scientific and Cultural Organization). (2009) *International Technical Guidance on Sexuality Education: An Evidence-Informed Approach for Schools* (Vol. 1 and 2). Paris: Teachers and Health Educators.

UNICEF. (2002) *Young People and HIV/AIDS: Opportunity in Crisis* UNICEF. New York: UNICEF.

UNICEF. (2005) *Unite for Children. Unite Against AIDS A Call to Action: Children, the Missing Face of AIDS*. New York: UNICEF.

UNICEF. (2007) *Progress for Children: A World Fit For Children Statistical Review* (No. 6). New York: UNICEF.

UNICEF. (2013) *Towards an AIDS-Free Generation Children and AIDS. Sixth Stocktaking Report*. New York: UNICEF.

United Nations Development Programme. (2003) *South African Human Development Report 2003*, Oxford: Oxford University Press.

Valdiserri, R. O. (2002) 'HIV-Related Stigma: An Impediment to Public Health'. *American Journal of Public Health*, 92: 341–342.

van Dyk, A. (2008). 'Perspectives of South African School Children on HIV/AIDS, and the Implications for Education Programmes'. *African Journal of AIDS Research*, 7(1): 79–93.

Vance, C. S. (ed). (1984) *Pleasure and Danger: Exploring Female Sexuality*. New York: Routledge & Kegan Paul Books.

Walker, J. (2004) 'Parents and Sex Education: Looking Beyond "the Birds and the Bees" '. *Sex Education*, 4(3): 239–254.

Walker, J. & Milton, J. (2006) 'Teachers' and Parents' Roles in the Sexuality Education of Primary School Children: A Comparison of Experiences in Leeds, UK and in Sydney, Australia'. *Sex Education*, 6(4): 415–428.

Walkerdine, V. (2004) 'Development Psychology and the Study of Childhood', in M. Kehily (ed) *An Introduction to Childhood Studies* (pp. 112–124). Buckingham: Open University Press.

Watney, S. (1991) 'School's Out', in D. Fuss (ed) *Inside/Out: Lesbian Theories, Gay Theories* (pp. 387–404). London: Routledge.

Weeks, J. (1986) *Sexuality*. London: Routledge.

Weeks, J. (2000) *Making Sexual History*. Cambridge: Polity Press.

WHO (World Health Organization). (2013) *Global and Regional Estimates of Violence Against Women: Prevalence and Health Effects of Intimate Partner Violence and Non Partner Sexual Violence*. Geneva: WHO.

Wood, K. & Jewkes, R. (2001). ' "Dangerous" Love: Reflections on Violence Among Xhosa Township Youth', in R. Morrell (ed) *Changing Men in Southern Africa* (pp. 317–336). Pietermaritzburg: University of Natal Press.

Wood, K., Lambert, H. & Jewkes, R. (2007) 'Showing Roughness in a Beautiful Way'. *Medical Anthropology Quarterly*, 21(3): 277–300.

Wood, L. & Rolleri, L. A. (2014) 'Designing an Effective Sexuality Education Control Themselves': Teachers' Beliefs and Attitudes Towards Young People's Sexual and Curriculum for Schools: Lessons Gleaned From the South(ern) African Literature'. *Sex Education: Sexuality, Society and Learning*, 14(5): 525–542.

# Index

www.ingramcontent.com/pod-product-compliance
Ingram Content Group UK Ltd.
Pitfield, Milton Keynes, MK11 3LW, UK
UKHW020429010325
455677UK00029B/1075